GLOSSECTOMEE
SPEECH REHABILITATION

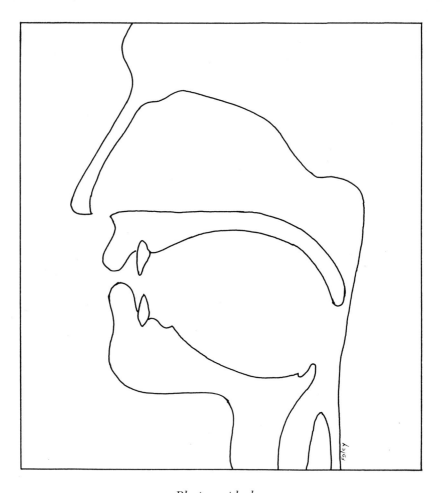

Photographs by

Toy T. Garris

Chief, Medical Illustration Service
Veterans Administration Hospital
St. Louis, Missouri

Illustrations by

Frank Foley

Medical Artist, Medical Illustration Service
Veterans Administration Hospital
St. Louis, Missouri

GLOSSECTOMEE
SPEECH REHABILITATION

By

MADGE SKELLY, Ph.D.

Chief, Audiology and Speech Pathology Service
Veterans Administration Hospital
Clinical Professor of Communication Disorders
St. Louis University
St. Louis, Missouri

With Chapters by

ROBERT C. DONALDSON, M.D.

Associate Chief, Surgical Service
Veterans Administration Hospital
Instructor in Surgery
Washington University School
of Medicine
St. Louis, Missouri

RITA SOLOVITZ FUST, M.A.

Speech Pathologist
Veterans Administration Hospital
St. Louis, Missouri

and a Foreword by

Barbara J. Seelye, Ph.D.

Professor and Chairman, Department of Communication Disorders
St. Louis University
St. Louis, Missouri

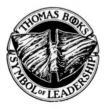

CHARLES C THOMAS · PUBLISHER
Springfield · Illinois · U.S.A.

Published and Distributed Throughout the World by
CHARLES C THOMAS · PUBLISHER
Bannerstone House
301–327 East Lawrence Avenue, Springfield, Illinois, U.S.A.

© *1973, by* CHARLES C THOMAS · PUBLISHER
ISBN 0–398–02706–4
Library of Congress Catalog Card Number: 72–88455

With THOMAS BOOKS *careful attention is given to all details of manufacturing and design. It is the Publisher's desire to present books that are satisfactory as to their physical qualities and artistic possibilities and appropriate for their particular use.* THOMAS BOOKS *will be true to those laws of quality that assure a good name and good will.*

Printed in the United States of America
K–8

To

KENNETH COLE, M.D.

*who assisted the birth
and inspired the growth
of the Cochran Speech Clinic
at St. Louis Veterans
Administration Hospital*

FOREWORD

EVERYONE FAMILIAR with the adventure movies of the thirties, forties and early fifties is acquainted with the dramatic moment when, in the presence of the assembled Court, the King declares with anger, "Take him thither! Tear out his tongue!" The poor messenger who brought the news of the lost battle is then dragged from the room to be forever silenced. Literature has always described the tragic treatment of slaves, bodyguards privy to state secrets, etc., who were silenced by this most dramatic and punitive of treatments. Perhaps it has been the long tradition of silencing the individual through tongue removal which has contributed to the lack of creative research and clinical endeavor with the glossectomee. The reports of work with the glossectomee which were published were based upon small numbers of cases, with little systemized study of the effects and results of the therapeutic attempts.

Such omission of treatment and/or therapeutic endeavor with the glossectomee has been excused at times by the rationale, "We just don't get those patients." This may be a justifiable explanation, since, as the authors found, few of the glossectomees have been referred to speech pathologists for rehabilitation. Certainly, with the publication of this carefully researched clinical book, information will now be available for the physician, clinician and family of the glossectomee, so that referral can become as routine as with formerly considered "impossible" speech cases.

Dr. Skelly and her associates have made a valuable contribution to clinical literature not only because they have analyzed and systematized a therapeutic approach to speech rehabilitation of the individual whose tongue has been removed but also because the results of their years of study and analysis challenge the imagination of the professional research worker as well as the clinician. As any basic work in an area stimulates further growth and refinement of understanding and technique, this volume opens the door for medical and clinical study in further depth. All too often research opens new pathways of thought but offers no direct clinical application to the practicing clinician who has neither the time, money, expertise nor number of case types to develop clinical technique based upon the results of the research. This book will be welcomed by practicing clinicians as an addition to their library which not only tells them what the problem is but also what can be done about the problem. It is an example of the contribution to the professional body of information which can be made and should be made by the clinically orientated professional who has an interest in research.

As outlined in the preface, pilot work with the project was developed and reported before the larger study was formalized. The reception of the pilot study results was enthusiastic and a definitive indicator of the desire for and need for elaborated information. Although some may differ with various points made, particularly in the details of therapeutic development, there are few who can disagree with the results—93 people who can speak and speak well.

It is always a matter of pride to watch and indirectly participate in the professional development of creative clinicians, especially when one has taught the Chief of Service, Dr. Skelly, in the classroom and clinic. It is a matter of extraordinary pride when the former student surpasses the teacher in some area of interest. It is a matter of indescribable pride when the former student contributes to the professional body of literature a work which one believes will become a basic text in the field.

BARBARA J. SEELYE

PREFACE

THE MAJOR purpose of this book is to provide currently available information on speech rehabilitation of the total glossectomee. Almost every laryngectomee receives some voice and speech training. The American Cancer Society reports that for each three laryngectomees there are two glossectomees. Yet the latter have had little or no speech rehabilitation developed to help them achieve usable oral communication.

The book is divided into three major sections. The first provides background on the problem. Recent summaries of cancer incidence, types, etiologies and prevention measures are included. The surgeon describes preoperative and postoperative phases of patient care, pointing out the need for speech rehabilitation. The literature to date on such rehabilitation is reviewed. Part Two reports the exploratory studies conducted by the authors. Part Three describes the techniques and procedures developed from the experimental work for patient treatment.

The clinical portion is approximately half of the total volume. It includes a wide range of general and specific methods and materials for use with the compensatory phoneme problems resulting from such highly individualized surgery. The illustrations vividly contrast the normal and compensatory production of each glossal phoneme.

Extensive testing procedures are described with their rationale. Tests forms permitting deductions for therapy planning may be reproduced. Forms for summarization of surgical and other patient information appear in the Appendix. A behavioral analysis of Leiter scores is among them. Nonglossal word and sentence lists as well as word and sentence lists for each of the glossal phonemes also are provided.

The book owes much to the assistance of a great many people as well as to the opportunities the senior author has enjoyed of presenting the slowly evolving techniques at various workshops and conferences. Among these were the International Triennial Congress of Logopedics and Phoniatrics at Buenos Aires in 1971, the Head and Neck Cancer Conference at University of Miami School of Medicine in 1969 and 1970, the Annual Meeting of the American Speech and Hearing Association in 1968 and 1969, as well as presentations at Duke University School of Medicine, University of Mississippi, University of Georgia, Washington University School of Medicine, St. Louis University School of Medicine, several state Cancer Societies and a wide variety of interdisciplinary professional meetings at hospitals and with state and federal personnel serving the handicapped.

Probably the most important thing to be said for the book and for the five years' work that went into its preparation is that it demonstrates that the tongueless patient can learn to talk intelligibly and that it provides directives that have enabled a great many glossectomees to accomplish what has been regarded for centuries as an impossibility. The search of the literature has revealed no other work or text presenting any helpful organized plan of speech rehabilitation for these patients based on experience with an adequate number of subjects. If this book interests surgeons and speech pathologists in the speech problems of glossectomees, provides some assistance to the speech clinician in treating the problem and provokes further inquiry in clinical research for building upon and improving upon that which has been developed here, the best hopes of the authors will be fulfilled and more glossectomee patients will be restored to a useful level of oral communication.

ACKNOWLEDGMENTS

THE AUTHORS gratefully acknowledge the cooperation of the American Cancer Society, Funk and Wagnalls and Bernard Glemser, the *American Journal of Surgery* and the *Journal of Speech and Hearing Disorders,* all of whom gave permission for quotations or reprinting of their published materials.

Without the generous, selfless devotion of two particular people the Speech Clinic would not have been organized to do the work: Dr. Kenneth Cole, who was at that time Chief of the Physical Medicine and Rehabilitation Service, and Miss Lillian Carney, who has been the Chief of the Occupational Therapy Section for a number of years. Without the surgical skill, human empathy and devoted patient care provided by Dr. Robert C. Donaldson, the project would never have been initiated.

Special recognition is due a number of people who participated in the clinical research projects and contributed to the articles upon which two of the chapters are based: Dr. Armand Brodeur, M.D., Chief of the Radiology Service at Cardinal Glennon Hospital, Francis X. Paletta, M.D., Professor of Plastic Surgery at St. Louis University School of Medicine, and Diane Spector, M.A., who served as a speech clinician during the initial phases of the project.

Dr. Albert Knox, Chief of the Audiology and Speech Pathology Service at the Kansas City Veterans Administration Hospital, gave generously of his time and advice and provided the opportunity to print the sonagrams of the early units. Nathaniel Levin, M.D., of the Otolaryngology Service at the University of Miami Medical School provided both encouragement and opportunity for discussion and experimentation. Dr. Elizabeth Carrow, editor of the *Journal of Speech and Hearing Disorders,* with her pertinent and constructive criticism, improved the reporting skills of the team.

xi

Mr. David Anton, Director of the St. Louis Veterans Hospital, its Chief of Staff, Dr. Ralph Biddy, its Associate Chief of Staff for Research and Education, Dr. Francis Carey, all provided encouragement and support. Directors of the two affiliated training programs, Dr. Barbara Seelye of St. Louis University and Sr. Dorothea Buchanan of Fontbonne College, afforded opportunity for valuable discussion of the work in progress. Diana Townsend, Lorraine Schinsky, Larry Warren and Randall Smith, speech pathologists at the St. Louis Veterans Administration, assisted in improving both the therapeutic techniques and the reporting of them.

The intelligent, tireless and meticulous work of Mrs. Mary Loafman, secretary of the Audiology and Speech Pathology Service at the St. Louis Veterans Administration Hospital is very much appreciated. Without her, this book would be still unwritten.

All of these people join with me in gratitude and admiration of the cheerful, patient cooperation afforded the team by the glossectomee patients who participated.

Royalties from this book have been assigned to the research program of the American Cancer Society.

MADGE SKELLY

CONTENTS

xiii

GLOSSECTOMEE
SPEECH REHABILITATION

PART ONE

BACKGROUND

Chapter I

THE PROBLEM

INCIDENCE

THE AMERICAN CANCER SOCIETY in its *Cancer Facts and Figures* (1971) stated that five per cent of all cancers occur in the oral cavity. It predicted that mouth cancer will be diagnosed in about 15,000 persons and will cause approximately 7,000 deaths in the U. S. in a calendar year at the present time. Carcinoma of the tongue is ranked as the second most frequent form of oral cancer.

In age-adjusted death rates for all cancer sites per 100,000 population around the world, Portugal showed the lowest rate at 108 for males and 83 for females. Scotland was listed as having the highest with 199 for males and 126 for females. The United States reported 138 for males and 103 for females. An important rehabilitation aspect of the cancer statistics was demonstrated by comparison of total United States cancer death figures for 1969 (325,000) with the almost double incidence of new cases (615,000) in that year. Only heart disease outranked cancer in leading causes of death. With the total number of deaths at 1,863,149, cancer was listed as the cause for 303,736. While these figures place the United States eighteenth from the highest in terms of all cancer sites, it ranks sixth for oral cancers in males and tenth in females.

PREDISPOSING FACTORS

Chronic irritation of long standing has been widely recognized as one of the most frequently present predisposing factors in the development of cancer. Irritation of the oral mucosa may have a variety of causes. Cancer may be due to several sources of irritation. Over-exposure to the weather and sunlight is a significant causative factor in cancer of the lower lip. Sun, wind, and dust, with lack of normal atmospheric moisture, produce an almost

5

constant dryness of the labial mucosa. The use of snuff in some geographical areas has a part in the etiology of cancer in the inferior gingiva and in buccal mucosa. "The chronicity of the irritant is more important than its nature," Martin (1940).

Chronic inflammatory conditions such as syphilitic glossitis and stomatitis seem to be predisposing to cancer. These latter may be due to a nutritional deficiency such as avitaminosis B. Tobacco and alcohol, when taken together with the resulting deficiencies in vitamin and protein intake and the subsequent liver damage, may play a part in producing the cancer. Long-standing trauma to the oral mucosa by sharp, defective teeth or ill-fitting dentures is also considered by some authorities to be a contributing cause of oral cancer.

PRECANCEROUS LESIONS

Leukoplakia occurs as a tissue response to chronic irritation. It is often found to precede or to be associated with cancer. Among other chronic lesions which sometimes become malignant are papillomas, fissures and ulcers. These lesions, however, are not always necessarily precancerous.

Leukoplakia, which appears as a white thickening, may occur anywhere on the mucosa of the oral cavity. The surface of this lesion may be smooth and thin, or it may be leathery and thick. Chronic fissures or ulcers may appear on a leukoplakic plaque. This lesion should be carefully observed for malignant change. Chronic labial fissures, particularly those in the midline of the lower lip, characteristically undergo repeated sequences of healing and breakdown. As a result of chronic irritation, they may eventually become malignant.

Papillomas, polyps and benign tumors occurring on the mucosa of the cheek or tongue are very often subjected to trauma by the teeth. Such lesions rarely become malignant. Chronic ulcers of the mouth, however, particularly those arising from such trauma may become malignant. If such ulcers do not heal within a few weeks after the removal of the irritating agent, they should be regarded with suspicion. Clinical signs of chronicity, tumefaction, ulceration and induration are highly significant precancerous alerts.

CANCERS OF THE ORAL CAVITY

Lip

Carcinoma of the lip in the vermilion zone is the most common of all oral cancers. In the early stage, it appears as an almost undetectable small swelling or induration. As it increases in size, it may grow outward as a fungating, ulcerated mass, or it may remain as a small, sharply punched-out ulcerative area with marked infiltration into the tissues of the lip. It may be diagnosed as herpes simplex, chancre, hyperkeratosis, or leukoplakia.

Buccal Mucosa

Cancer of the buccal mucosa appears most frequently in the middle third of the cheek. It is a fungating, papillary type of lesion. It frequently occurs in an area of leukoplakia. The margins of the lesion are rolled and indurated. Some of the lesions may be small, crateriform ulcers with elevated margins. Diagnosis will differentiate aphthous stomatitis, ulceromembranous stomatitis, traumatic ulcers, or tuberculous and syphilitic lesions.

Floor of the Mouth

A small nodule or ulceration may become a papillomatous type of growth or an ulcerous lesion with indurated margins. Although leukoplakia in this area is less common than elsewhere in the oral cavity, the lesion often arises in any existing area of leukoplakia. Those in the anterior two thirds of the floor of the mouth are frequently less malignant than more posterior lesions. Metastases to the cervical lymph nodes occur early. Examination will distinguish Vincent's angina, simple inflammatory ulcers, or obstruction and swelling of submandibular or sublingual ducts and glands. Cancer of the floor of the mouth is closely allied to cancer of the tongue because of the juxtaposition of these sites, with probable common etiology of malignant tumors.

The Palate

Cancer may occur in either the hard or the soft palate. The lesion is usually the epidermoid, squamous cell type, although it is somewhat glandular. It may appear as a shallow, punched-out ulcer with rolled indurated margins, or it may be a papillary growth with a wide base. The adenocarcinomatous lesion is a nodular tumor which may eventually ulcerate. The early detection of palatal cancer is particularly urgent because advanced growth may cause permanent dysfunction by perforating the palate and putting the nasal and oral cavities in communication. Differential diagnosis isolates a papilloma, torus palatinus and mixed tumors of the minor salivary glands.

The Gingiva

Early signs of gingival carcinoma include mucosal thickenings, erosions and advanced leukoplakic plaques. These lesions are rarely seen in the anterior portion of the mouth. They usually arise in the molar and bicuspid regions. The growth characteristically spreads along the gum, becoming nodular, warty or papillary. The spread is usually extensive before ulceration. The gums, being intermediate in position between vestibule and oral cavity proper, have many routes of contiguous spread, including the chin, floor of the mouth, gingivolingual sulcus and the tongue. Infiltration of the mandible may readily follow. In addition to bone destruction by direct cancer infiltration, bone changes due to pressure erosion may occur. Superiorly the lesion may even extend to the nasal septum, floor of the nasal cavity, and the maxillary antrum. Inflammatory hyperplastic gingivitis, traumatic lesions, subperiosteal abscess and giant cell granuloma may be differentiated.

The Tongue

The tongue occupies the major area of the floor of the mouth. It consists of two parts, the body and the root. Anatomically, the root of the tongue refers to that portion of the organ which is directly related to the floor of the mouth. It is the true muscular base. The body has an inferior surface which is chiefly related to the floor of the mouth, where it receives the intrinsic musculature. The inferior lateral portions, however, lie free in the oral cavity. They form the medial limit of the gingivolingual sulci. This free inferior surface presents as the frenulum in the midline.

On the dorsum of the tongue, the most conspicuous gross anatomical structures are the circumvallate papillae, each surrounded by a fossae. These are arranged in the shape of an inverted V at the junction of the oral and pharyngeal parts of the tongue. The portion of the tongue behind the circumvallate papillae is termed the base of the tongue. It is considered part of the oropharynx. Many authors currently designate this base as the posterior one third of the tongue, while others using this fractional locator mean the posterior third of the mobile tongue. Confusion may arise unless mobile or base is designated. A lateral border of the oral portion of the tongue may be defined at the junction of the inferior surface and the dorsum. This lateral border, particularly its posterior portion, is the most frequent site of cancer involving the oral tongue.

Carcinoma of the tongue has been consistently reported as the second most frequent form of oral cancer. These lesions are commonly preceded by leukoplakia. Most tongue cancers appear on the lateral surfaces, although they may arise on the superior, or inferior surfaces. Generally, the more posterior the lesion, the more malignant it becomes. It may be the ulcerative, infiltrating type or the fungating, papillary type of lesion. A third type of malignant lesion, the fissure type, may occur at the junction of the lateral base of the tongue and the anterior tonsillar pillar. This lesion may be easily missed on examination. Differential diagnosis includes aphthous stomatitis, ulceromembranous ulcers, traumatic ulcers, leukoplakia, mucous patch or gumma syphilis, tuberculous ulcers, geographic or hairy tongue, or median rhomboid glossitis.

Tumors of the buccal portion of the tongue may extend mucosally or submucosally in a posterior direction to invade the oropharynx. In a lateral direction, they may invade the floor of the mouth. If the tumor extends deep into the muscle, it may spread along the muscle planes to infiltrate the whole tongue. The hyoid bone, the mandible and styloid process may be invaded, thus affecting the intrinsic muscles of the tongue. Metastatic cells may pass freely from any part of the tongue to lymph nodes on *both* sides of the neck. Metastases to cervical nodes occur more frequently from tongue cancer than from any other intraoral primary site. Even distant metastases are not uncommon. The lung and liver are most frequently involved.

SYMPTOMS

Since early identification is highly related to successful alleviation, speech pathologists should join the physicians and dentists in the cancer symptom alert. Early warning signs are easily discernible but often ignored. Most of the early symptoms are painless. Although none of the following signs necessarily indicate the presence of cancer, they warrant immediate medical attention:

1. Unusual bleeding or discharge.
2. A lump or swelling of the lips, gum, tongue, cheek, palate, tonsils, neck.
3. A sore or ulceration that does not heal within two weeks.
4. White scaly areas inside the mouth with numbness or loss of feeling.

PREVENTION

In order to prevent cancer of the mouth, it is advisable to avoid or correct conditions which may encourage it.

1. Prolonged exposure to strong sunlight should be avoided. The lips should be covered with a protective cream if exposure is unavoidable.
2. Teeth or dentures that irritate the surrounding tissue should have the immediate attention of the dentist.
3. Any lump, scaly area or white spot on the lips or in the mouth which lasts longer than two weeks should be seen by a physician.
4. Mouth cancer is sometimes preceded by unhealthy mucous membranes in the mouth, pharynx and esophagus, caused by dietary deficiencies. Information is readily available from many free sources concerning items and proportions of foods necessary for a balanced diet.
5. High heat is an irritant to living tissue. Frequent use of excessively hot foods or drinks should be avoided.
6. Cleanliness is always important in disease prevention. Thorough and frequent brushing of the teeth is desirable as well as a regular annual dental checkup.

7. Mouth cancers are more frequently found in heavy drinkers of alcohol than in the general population.
8. There is considerable evidence that irritation from the use of tobacco is highly related causally to cancer.

Since 1959, the American Cancer Society has carried on an extensive Cancer Prevention Study, with some 68,000 investigators in 1,121 counties interviewing 1,079,000 men and women over the age of thirty. Over 18 scientific papers have been published, based on the results of early followups. The last followups have been completed (1969), and 98.5 per cent of originally enrolled persons have been traced. On the data from this project, one report on life expectancy in relation to cigarette smoking showed that 25-year-old men who smoke two packs a day have a life expectancy of 8.3 years less than a comparable group of men who have never smoked.

Bernard Glemser, in *Man Against Cancer,* writes:

The American Cancer Society and the Canadian Cancer Society and the British Empire Cancer Fund and the French National League Against Cancer and the Japanese Cancer Society and all the other organizations around the world are concerned about malignant disease. There are many causes of lung cancer; asbestos dust is known to be implicated, and so are oil mists used on certain machine tools. Workers in the chromate industry are more susceptible than the general population; and uranium miners, exposed to radioactive ores, respond predictably with a high rate of lung tumors. But the principal cause of lung cancer is smoking of cigarettes, although other factors may be involved.

In the United States, sixty thousand people now die in a year as a result of lung cancer, and of these fifty-four thousand will be cigarette smokers.

A safe cigarette is no more possible than safe cynanide. Every time a more effective filter has been devised it has been necessary to strengthen the flavor of the tobacco in some manner, by using coarser cuts or different blends, so that the fastidious smoker can taste the carcinogens he is taking into his respiratory system. Otherwise, cigarette manufacturers have learned from long and costly experience, the fastidious smoker feels he is being robbed of something infinitely precious and he will immediately switch to another brand. A safer cigarette today would probably arouse such widespread consumer resistance that it would almost certainly be followed by a far more dangerous cigarette tomorrow; and the truth of this statement is shown by the constant increase in the length of cigarettes, from the so called normal or regular size (which were carcinogenic enough) to king sized (which are ten or fifteen per cent more carcinogenic) to still longer kinds (which are proportionately more carcinogenic than their predecessors).

There is little hope that anything can be done about this particular insanity. It may be indeed part of some intricate particular evolutionary process, whereby at a time when populations are increasing rather too rapidly for comfort, nature supplies the means . . . an insatiable craving for a destructive toxin . . . to check the rate of increase. Lung cancer, cancer of the bladder, emphysema, and heart disease, all circulatory diseases such as Buerger's disease: all arise from tobacco tars and nicotine, all serve to reduce the population. Even in Japan and India, where lung cancer was unknown until recently, it is now known only too well; and today there are no unshaded areas left on the lung cancer map of the world.

It is preventable. It need not happen. *It really is preventable.*

SPEECH PATHOLOGY

The profession of speech pathology has consistently, from its inception, devoted a sizeable portion of its clinical and research efforts to the voice and speech problems of laryngectomees, most of whom have had the larynx excised as a consequence of cancer. In large hospital-based clinics, often from 25 to 40 per cent of the total patient load may be laryngectomees. In contrast, only minimal research and clinical effort has been directed toward the speech and voice problems of patients with cancer surgery of other oral, facial and pharyngeal areas. The Cancer Society reported for 1966 an incidence of 2800 new cases of cancer of the larynx. It is pertinent, in view of the wide attention to speech problems of the laryngectomee, that the same report indicated 1725 glossectomees, most of whom are not referred to or examined by a speech pathologist for rehabilitation. A large proportion of the glossectomee population have additional surgical alterations such as hemimandibulectomy. Some are also laryngectomees. The skills of modern plastic surgery have extended the life span of many cancer patients. As a result, an increasing number of persons who have lost portions of the mechanisms for mastication, deglutition, phonation and articulation are left with consequent severe disabilities. Laryngectomy causes the loss of voice. Glossectomy prevents normal articulation of the speech sounds. If a portion of the jaw is removed, additional dental and mandibular problems ensue. Mandibular excursion and labial movement may be limited. Dysphagia or regurgitation may occur. The palate is often included in the resection or suffers scarring contraction or loss of soft palate motility. Hyperrhinolalia will distort any existing speech, so that intelligibility will be negligible.

If the individual experiences the usual gradual diminution of hearing acuity with age, an additional problem complicates the necessary auditory self-monitoring of speech attempt. When the larynx is removed, the ensuing aphonia is compensated by development of esophageal voice or by use of the electrolarynx. Voice without articulation, however, is inadequate for intelligible communication. If additional portions of the oral and pharyngeal mechanisms are excised, few organs remain for compensatory function. Principally because the speech distortions consequent to total tongue excision have been largely regarded as irreversible, little has been done to assist speech rehabilitation of total glossectomees.

Chapter II

PHASES OF PATIENT CARE
ROBERT C. DONALDSON

PREOPERATIVE, OPERATIVE AND POSTOPERATIVE

TOTAL GLOSSECTOMY for cancer involving 50 per cent or more of the tongue has been slow to gain wide acceptance in the treatment of this disease because of the commonly accepted, potentially grim postoperative outlook. Nevertheless, the operative approach is the only method of treatment with an appreciable three-year survival rate (Donaldson *et al.,* 1968). This same study shows individual patients with postoperative survival of 10, 9½, 8½, 7 and 4½ years.

A wide range of potential postoperative complications, both physical and psychological, confronts both patient and doctor at the time the patient appears for treatment of cancer involving more than one half of the tongue. How successfully will this patient swallow and talk? Will he be employable? What are his chances for aspiration of food into the trachea with the consequent threat of pneumonia? How will the deformity of the face due to loss of one-half the mandible affect his relations with family, friends and strangers? Will he be understood over the telephone? Will he be able to adjust to eating at the same table as family and friends when he uses a bulb syringe to place the liquid diet in his mouth? And last, but not least, what are his chances of cure? Without a doubt, total glossectomy with or without the removal of the larynx represents to the patient the ultimate in personal disability and to the speech pathologist the ultimate challenge to develop useful communication for the patient.

The presence of any advanced, associated disease of any other organ system could contraindicate the oral surgery. Also, the cancer can spread locally beyond the tongue to the lateral and posterior pharynx and into the neck and to the base of the skull and as a result be nonresectable. Prognostically, only one sign is of any predictive value: absence of microscopic cancer in the lymph nodes. The prognosis is only half as good if the cancer has spread to the cervical lymph nodes.

Preparation of the patient to accept surgery involves a biopsy for tissue diagnosis and a complete physical examination including an indirect and direct laryngoscopy to determine the extent of the disease. It is of the utmost importance to determine preoperatively if the larynx can be preserved. After the tissue diagnosis and extent of the disease have been determined, the entire situation is explained to the patient in a frank manner, leaving nothing for the patient to guess about. Thus he is prepared to meet the challenge of postoperative rehabilitation.

Two or three days later, a second conference is held. This time the patient's nearest relative, usually a wife, is included. Both are encouraged to ask questions. Every attempt is made to answer frankly all questions regarding postoperative problems.

Ideally the patient should be introduced to another patient who has had a total glossectomy and be allowed to ask him questions and observe how well he speaks. The patient is then referred to the speech pathologist for preoperative recording of his voice patterns. This serves also as an introduction to the methods of speech rehabilitation to be used following surgery.

At this point, a date is set for the operation and the patient is asked to sign the operative permit. The patient may expect to be hospitalized approximately one week prior to surgery and from two to six weeks postoperatively.

Curative cancer surgery requires that the surgeon remove not only the primary lesion but also the area to which cancer is most likely to spread. Wide margins of normal tissue must also be excised. Tissue to be removed will include lymph nodes of the neck, platysma, sternocleidomastoid muscle, internal jugular vein, omohyoid muscle, anterior and posterior bellies of the digastric muscle, stylohyoid muscle, submaxillary salivary gland, tail of the parotid gland, all branches of the external carotid artery ex-

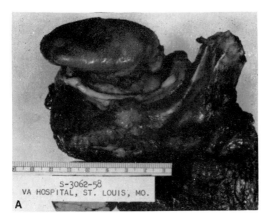

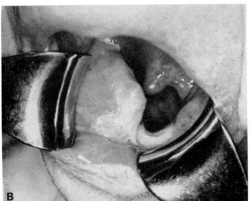

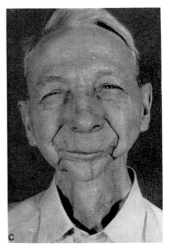

Figure 1. A, Cancer involving the base of the tongue and floor of mouth laterally and anteriorly across the midline. B, Postoperative appearance of mouth with skin graft in place. C, Appearance of patient nine years postoperatively. (Figure 1 photographs courtesy *American Journal of Surgery*).

cept the superior thyroid, one-half of the mandible, the entire tongue and if needed, the epiglottis, hyoid bone and even occasionally the larynx.

Nerves severed will include the accessory, ansa hypoglossi, cervical sensory, mandibular branch of the facial and the hypoglossal. Every effort is made to preserve the vagus, superior laryngeal, cervical sympathetic and phrenic nerves and the brachial plexus. Other structures to be preserved are the common and internal carotid arteries.

Some glossectomy patients are edentulous. When teeth are present they are usually in an advanced state of decay. Poor dental hygiene goes hand in hand with malignancy of the mouth. A satisfactory bone graft replacement becomes almost impossible because of lack of tissue to cover it. As yet, no way has been found to construct a useful lower denture for the total glossectomee. Upper dentures are helpful from the cosmetic standpoint and are always provided for the edentulous patient at a suitable point in his rehabilitation program.

Most operative wounds are healed within 10 to 14 days if no infection occurs. All patients receive antibiotics before and after the operation to help guard against infection. Nasogastric suction is maintained for 48 hours to eliminate the possibility of early vomiting and aspiration. Postoperatively, a suction catheter is maintained beneath the skin covering the site of the neck dissection for three to nine days to prevent accumulation of lymph.

The tracheostomy tube which is routinely inserted at the operation is removed when a free airway via the glottis is demonstrated to exist by total obstruction of the tube with a cork (21st to 30th postoperative day) . The tracheostomy closes spontaneously within 48 to 72 hours after removal of the tracheostomy tube. The patient is encouraged to attempt to swallow water administered via a bulb syringe.

When the patient no longer aspirates water into his trachea, the nasogastric feeding tube is discarded. The patient is then given a liquid diet prepared with the aid of a food blender. A high-calorie, high-protein diet plus liquid vitamins is recommended. The patient is told to put the foods he likes best and usually eats into a blender, in milk preferably, with the liquid vitamins added. The blender diet should pour easily. Each patient will need to experiment to find the consistency which he can swallow best. The majority of patients report routine acceptance by the family of this method of eating. Solid foods and medicine in pill form are forever forbidden for the total glossectomee because of the danger of aspiration pneumonia.

When the superior laryngeal nerve is severed at the operation because of the extent of the cancer, the mucosa about the glottis becomes anesthetic. Since this patient then is unable to sense the presence of food or liquid, he rarely learns to swallow without aspiration. He may require insertion of a short nasoesophageal feeding tube at each meal. Or he may acquire a permanent feeding gastrostomy. The solution of such swallowing problems is primarily the responsibility of the surgeon.

Donaldson (1968) has reported as follows on the act of swallowing in the normal and postoperative patient:

> The ability to swallow does not appear to be related to the presence or absence of the hyoid bone, or the intraoral skin graft. It is more likely related to preservation of the internal branch of the superior laryngeal nerve, the function of which is to provide sensory fibers to the epiglottis, aryepiglotic folds and to the larynx as low down as the vocal folds. . . . In the normal person, swallowing involves a combination of voluntary and involuntary movements of the muscles of the tongue, soft palate and pharynx. The involuntary portion of the act is triggered by way of the sensory fibers supplying the pharynx. Thus, stimulation of the hypopharynx with a cotton applicator will initiate a complete swallowing reflex. In the patient with total glossectomy, essentially all that is left of the swallowing mechanism is the involuntary part which, from our experience, is adequate for a good food intake. Because of the importance of the internal branch of the superior laryngeal nerve to the involuntary mechanism of swallowing, care must be taken to avoid injury to it when removing the hyoid bone. . . .
>
> The usual normal pharyngeal stage of swallowing involves successive contractions of the superior, middle and inferior constrictor muscles which rapidly force the bolus of food into the esophagus. An interesting alternative to this method of swallowing occurs with certain patients who learn voluntarily to relax the cricopharyngeus muscle and pour liquids into the esophagus without making any use of the constrictors.

Drooling of saliva from the mouth is a common problem with considerable psychological and social drawbacks. Because of anatomical considerations, drooling is more of a problem when only part of the tongue is removed. The total glossectomee rarely drools, although he will tend unavoidably to spit saliva as he tries to talk. Reduction in the amount of saliva in the mouth by staged ligation of the ducts from both parotid glands has done much to correct this problem, although it is not done routinely when excision is total. The patient can rinse his mouth and gargle for oral hygiene at will.

Rehabilitation in communication starts on the first postoperative day. Since most patients can read and write, this is their first form of communication. A great morale builder is to demonstrate to the patient whose larynx remains intact that he can vocalize. A gloved finger is placed over the tracheostomy tube during expiration and the patient is asked to say "okay." The patient actually says "ohay" which will sound reasonably like a normal vocalization of this word.

Speech rehabilitation may start prior to the removal of the tracheostomy tube, perhaps as early as the tenth postoperative day. It should continue until the speech pathologist believes the patient has achieved his best possible speech.

These patients can never be completely separated from the medical environment which has cured them of their cancer and enabled them to achieve maximal rehabilitation. They need periodic examination for reappearance of cancer which can be further treated with chemotherapy or radiation therapy. This monthly examination continues indefinitely. During the first five years, it is to detect recurrence of the initial lesion. During the following five to ten years, it is to detect early the new primary which occurs in approximately one third of the five-year survivors.

The patients and their families need moral support and reassurance that all is well, both in terms of absence of disease and in terms of continued progress in rehabilitation. Most of these patients are retired. Employment opportunities are scarce. Usually self-employment is all that is available. Rarely a job at a domicillary as elevator operator is open.

These patients must not be shunned by society. They need to feel accepted and useful. A considerable mental uplift results when one of them is asked to encourage the next patient facing radical defunctioning and deforming surgery for cancer of the mouth. Usually this patient is proud to join his doctor as part of the team which deals with this form of cancer.

Chapter III

A HISTORY OF AGLOSSIA SPEECH REHABILITATION

INTRODUCTION

LINGUAL DEFORMITIES may be congenital, developmental, traumatic or surgical. Use of the terms "aglossia" and "dysglossia" are not always consistent in the literature but are classically defined as complete absence of the tongue in the former and alteration of the tongue in the latter. Other specific descriptive terms include macroglossia, microglossia, ankyloglossia, bifid or trifid tongue and tongue tie. Eating, chewing, swallowing and speaking difficulties may accrue from any of the former as well as from tongue paralyses, malfunctions due to scarring, or traumatic alterations resulting from war, highway, hunting or other accidents. One case on record was due to self-inflicted wounds. Cancer is the cause of the majority of the surgical excisions, total or partial. Glossectomy thus shares a common etiology with laryngectomy.

Laryngologists have consistently referred patients with surgical excision of the larynx for speech rehabilitation. In most VA Hospital Speech and Hearing Clinics, laryngectomees have usually comprised from 30 to 45 per cent of the caseload. Aside from a small percentage of brain tumor cases, the laryngectomees constituted the total surgical roster in speech, according to a 1969 and 1970 sampling at both the Head and Neck Cancer Conference at University of Miami Medical School and the Annual Meeting of the American Speech and Hearing Association. A like situation was reported at the International Congress of Logopedics and Phoniatrics at the University of Buenos Aires School of Medicine in 1971.

Concurrently, the American Cancer Society in its *Cancer Facts and Figures* (1969) and (1971) reveals that for every *three* patients with total extirpation of the larynx, there are *two* patients with total excision of the tongue. Yet very few of these patients have been referred for or have received any speech rehabilitation until recently.

THE PAST

Sixteenth to Nineteenth Century

The earliest therapeutic procedure in glossectomy has been attributed to Ambroise Paré (1510–1590). The illustrious French army surgeon was reputed to have designed a prosthesis for the tongueless. A round wooden plate held in the mouth and moved with the tongue stump was prescribed as an aid to articulation (Martin, 1940). A boy who had lost a very large portion of his tongue through gangrene has been described as quite intelligible by DeBelebat in 1630 in his book, *Aglossomography* (Luchsinger and Arnold, 1965). In 1718, Jussieu was reported in *Histoire de l'Academie des Sciences* as presenting in Paris a paper titled "Aglossia." It cited a case of congenital absence of the tongue, but the nine-year-old female subject was judged to have adequate intelligibility. In 1873, Edward Twistleton wrote "The Tongue Not Essential to Speech" which was published in London by John Murray. It recorded several cases in which the tongue had been either torn out or amputated. Yet some of the victims are reported as recovering usable speech.

Twentieth Century

First Decade

"A Case of Aglossia" in *Deutsche Medicinische Wochenschrift* by Kettner (1907) and a similar paper in the *New York Medical Record* by Seitz (1902) were cited by Goldstein (1940). These dealt with self development of somewhat useful speech by congenitally aglossic patients.

The Thirties

Froeschels, in 1933, contributed his useful therapeutic suggestion concerning the deglutinative process as a base for speech re-

habilitation exercises for many syndromes. Froeschels wrote that
he had many case reports of persons whose tongues were surgically
extirpated. He described some substitute adjustments of the other
oral structures to aid the individual to speak:

> The lower lip can be pressed against the incisors to substitute for
> the lingual sounds; the (s) and (f) can be made by blowing the air
> through the teeth or the protruded lips; the (r) can be made by
> quivering of the vocal cords or the uvula; the (l), (j), (i) and (e)
> can be produced by raising the floor of the mouth to approach the
> palate; the (k) and (g) can be formed by movements approximating
> the palatal arches.

The Forties

Keaster (1940) proposed that chewing and swallowing are more
difficult for the tongueless than speaking is.

"Speech Rehabilitation Following Excision of the Tip of the
Tongue" by Backus (1940) was an advance guard for a quicken-
ing of interest and acceleration of publication during the forties.
The paper described the case of a boy who lost his tongue tip but
who subsequently learned to speak again. Martin (1940), in the
American Journal of Surgery, published "The History of Lingual
Cancer." Professional speech clinicians became somewhat interested in the related speech problems of these patients but with
little published therapeutic result.

McEnerny and Gaines (1941) reported "tongue tie in infants
and children" as a tongue-related speech problem. Surgical severance of the frenum was frequently suggested in dysglossic speech
cases in the past. Even recently, tongue tie has been commonly
diagnosed by the layman as a cause of speech defects. These authors stated that they have never seen a tongue tie that needed to
be clipped. They reported that in over a thousand cases, only four
presented functionally shortened frenums. Even in this group,
there was no high correlation with speech problems, as one case
exhibited no deviance whatever and a second showed only a slight
(r) variance which was shortly corrected. Greene (1945), in the
New York Journal of Medicine in "Anomalies of the Speech
Mechanism and Associated Voice and Speech Disorders," indi-

cated the comparative rarity of this relationship of tongue tie and speech deviance. In records of more than 40,000 cases, not more than 12 of functionally important restriction of the tongue by the frenum were noted. The implication was that false importance may have been attached to high lingual motility for speech.

Recurring attempts at prosthetic alleviation of the glossectomee's speech difficulties have been reported. Panconcelli Calzia (1943) evolved a dental prosthesis which extended the dental, alveolar and palatal points of apposition posteriorly. He hoped to assist the mutilated tongue stump to achieve adequate contact for consonant obstruction. "Relationship of Dentition to Speech," by Frowene and Moser (1944), contributed indirectly to the increasing therapeutic explorations of deviant function of the various articulators, including the tongue. They presented the case of a boy whose tongue had suffered severe lye burns, resulting in a narrow range of tongue movement. His speech recovery was described as satisfactory.

Eskew and Shepard (1949), in "Congenital Aglossia" in the *American Journal of Orthodontics,* reported on a 22-year-old Chinese patient with congenital aglossia who spoke, but with a definite "speech impediment": "In speaking, the buccinator muscles were very noticeable in their movement, as were the muscles of the floor of the mouth. Also in speaking there was a clearly audible intake of air and a tendency for saliva to escape from the corners of the mouth." The floor of this patient's mouth is described as smooth and flexible enough to be elevated as a tongue-like structure making contact with the incisal edges of the maxillary anterior teeth. The maxillary arch was malocclusal, constricted and triangular in form. For the [k], the speaker effected contact of the buccinators and the molars. The [t] was made similarly with some difference in breath stream control to differentiate it from [k]. "All vowels were produced clearly except (e) and (i)." It is probable that the authors mean the standard dictionary markings for the long vowels, rather than the IPA symbols, which would read [i] and [aɪ] for the above vowels.

Goldstein (1940), in *Laryngoscope,* published his "New Concepts of the Function of the Tongue" in which he reported the demonstration of three patients with surgical alteration of the tongue. Consistent with his other significant contributions in the field of speech and hearing, he made an imaginative extrapolation from this limited study. As part of his introduction, he wrote: "We have thought and taught empirically for over a century *that the tongue is absolutely essential* in the various consonant elements." After describing the progress of each patient, he commented that in the light of our long-held concepts concerning the primacy of the tongue in articulatory intelligibility, it should be impossible for these patients to produce understandable speech. They presented a challenge, he contended, to those concerned with speech production, phonetics and articulation. If indeed the tongue is so indispensable to speech, how were these tongueless speakers achieving their intelligibility? "In the light of modern acoustic principles and mechanics of speech, it is possible that much of the information concerning the physiological function of the tongue (for speech) has been developed with too much empiricism."

In the concluding section, he advised that "less attention should be given to empirically prescribed *positions* of the tongue." He suggested, instead, more emphasis on "modifications of the shape and size" of the oral cavity and its "accessories."

In the past three decades, this sage advice has appeared to have minimal impact, with a few notable exceptions. Prescribed positions of the tongue have continued to be deeply imbedded in the professional literature and pedagogy. A significant step forward was suggested by McDonald (1965) with the ballistic concept of movement in time and space between positions. The speech scientists, notably Perkell (1969) at Massachusetts Institute of Technology, demonstrated in research the validity of the concept of modification of the size and shape of the oral cavity as well as its openings, as a correlate of intelligibility. Perkell focused on the labial aperture and mandibular excursion as it affects the size and shape of the oral cavity. Sheldon (1964, 1965) made notable contributions on the action and importance of the pharyngeal port in the course of his extensive studies on cleft palate speech.

It is no derogation of Goldstein's contribution to point out that two of his three cases are partial, not total, glossectomees. Recent studies (described later in date order) demonstrated that any residual tongue fragment or stump can be utilized (by motivated patients who are not dysphagic) to produce moderately intelligible speech. The patients with total excision present the truly challenging problem.

The rather enthusiastic reporting of total intelligibility included in Goldstein's thesis is somewhat charactersitic of similar later reports where the rating has been by subjective assessment rather than objective measurement. These subjective ratings have usually been made by attending physicians or clinicians who were familiar with the patient's speech because of their involvement in his treatment. Another factor contaminating subjective ratings made at conference demonstrations lies in rehearsal by the patient of spoken materials to be presented. One who has drilled on prepared materials for a demonstration will undoubtedly create the impression of an intelligibility level considerably higher than that which is valid for him in the stresses of everyday communication.

In addition to the prepared question and answer conversation of his demonstration, the Goldstein paper provided specific illustration of the consonant cognates [t] and [d], [k] and [g] as well as [i] and also [n]. No mention is included of the cognates [s] and [z], or the [ŋ] or the two most difficult phonemes for the glossectomy: [r] and the cognates [θ] and [ð].

Even with the noted limitations and the very small number of cases (3), Goldstein's conclusions remain valid:

1. The tongue is not absolutely indispensable as an organ of articulate speech.
2. Various other parts of the mouth cavity may be utilized to replace it.
3. Understandable, fluent speech can be produced without a tongue.
4. Our knowledge of the physiology of the tongue as an organ of speech is subject to much needed revision.

Dr. Goldstein did not attempt to explain or describe what physiologic modifications provide the intelligibility of the patients he reports, nor did he claim any credit for the success achieved. Rather he attributed the progress in each case to the individual patient's own untutored efforts.

The Fifties

Kremer (1953) found that in cancer of the tongue requiring radical neck dissection, the speech was impaired in the early post-operative period but later improved. In 1955, Froeschels made an additional contribution to therapeutic techniques with the introduction of his "pushing" exercises. These have been best known for their clinical use in cases of dysphonia related to hypofunction. They have also proved highly profitable for the glossectomy patient in developing some control of drooling and alleviation of dysphagia when these conditions are present.

Bloomer, in the monumental work edited by Travis (1957), referred briefly to glossectomy among the "lingual deformities" which may adversely affect articulatory clarity. "Anyone of these abnormalities may affect speech, but the degree to which they may affect any individual case varies in accordance with factors other than the mere extent of the lingual deformity."

Herberman (1958) published a rehabilitation report on two patients following partial glossectomy: "The chief complaints of the patients in both instances were continued and uncontrolled salivation, inability to swallow solid foods, regurgitation of liquids through the nose, restriction or absence of movement of the lips, jaw, and neck and unintelligible speech." The paper indicated that at the time of discharge, [k], [g] and [ŋ] were "still absent" and that "the vowels were all nasalized." The summary noted that "therapy consisted primarily of increasing the facilities of chewing, sucking and swallowing."

Zimmerman presented an unpublished paper at the 1958 Annual Convention of the American Speech and Hearing Association. It reported clinical attempts at rehabilitation, resulting in minimal intelligibility progress in two cases.

Arnold, in Luchsinger and Arnold (1959) in the German edition and the revised edition (1965) in English, expressed the view that the aglossic patient can develop speech "either spontaneously or by systematic instruction." The missing sounds, he stated, are

developed gradually "by vicarious movement of the residual muscle stumps or remaining oral musculature."

Of the long vowels, he reported the phoneme [aɪ] as exhibiting
the greatest permanent limitation, although the others are also
distorted as follows:

[eɪ] sounds like [i]
[o] sounds like [oɪ]
[u] sounds like [j]
[i] between [i] and [oɪ]

Arnold suggested the following successful substitutions:

1. The [d], [t] and [n] were articulated clearly by elevating the
   lower lip behind the upper teeth as Goldstein had observed
   in 1940.
2. "Adroit" patients achieved a serviceable [s] by blowing
   through the teeth.
3. The [ʃ] was produced by modifying the [s] with protrusion
   of the lips.
4. The [g], [k] and [ŋ] were "articulated as pharyngeal sounds
   between the tongue residue or the epiglottis and the pharyngeal wall, although some patients made these sounds within
   the larynx similar to cleft palate speech."
5. A successful [r] was attributed to substitution of "the grunted
   vocal fry produced by slow subtonal vibrations of the vocal
   cords or ventricular folds."
6. The [l] was described as quite clear after a period of instruction, "even though the division of air stream cannot come
   about."

No indication was provided concerning the type of instruction
which successfully accomplished the substitutions. There was no
report of any consistent method of articulatory measurement of
pretherapy and posttherapy intelligibility, either subjective or
objective. Such assessment was undoubtedly made, and its in-
clusion would assist in more meaningful interpretation of the
report.

This author apparently assumed that in all dysglossic cases dentition remained intact and a flexible tongue stump was available.
Possibly the articulatory substitutions suggested were intended
to apply to cases of congenital aglossia or to those of tongue dam-

age caused by highway, industrial or war trauma rather than to
cases of surgical excision.

> The outlook for all dysglossic speech disorders resulting from injury
> of the tongue is generally very good. . . . Only the marked forms of
> acquired alterations of the tongue are important as true mechanical
> causes of dysglossic disorders of oral speech. . . . Direct injuries to
> the tongue were quite frequent during the two world wars. In times
> of peace, corresponding speech disorders are not rare after accidents
> or resulting from tongue operations such as for malignant tumors.

Arnold concluded that "loss of a considerable portion of the
tongue produces a very marked distortion of speaking."

Friedrich S. Brodnitz, in "Speech after Glossectomy" in *Current Problems in Phoniatrics and Logopedics* (1960), expressed
the same view: "Any event that alters the shape of the tongue or
interferes with lingual motility will create a severe articulatory
handicap." Since both Brodnitz and Arnold have an extensive
exposure to a large number of patients, as well as varieties of
etiologies among them, their agreement on the difficulty of aglossic speech constituted a significant contrast to the euphoric rather
than heuristic prognostications in the earlier literature, all made
from extremely limited samples.

Brodnitz pointed out the comparatively contemporary acceleration of surgical glossectomy for tongue cancer.

> Until recently, in the majority of these cases the loss of lingual tissue
> was due to accidental causes (chemical or electrical destruction,
> gunshot or shell wounds), or to infection or gangrene. With the
> development of radical surgical techniques in dealing with malig-
> nancies of the tongue and the floor of the mouth, more patients are
> seen after extensive surgery on the tongue and the other structures
> of the mouth. Removal of the tongue is often combined with radical
> dissection of the neck and/or resection of a part of the mandible. . . .

He cautioned that in the latter case, the interruption of the motor
and/or sensory fibers may also impair control of the lips. (In view
of the emphasis on labial substitution in the previous literature
on this problem, this is an important factor to be considered in
both diagnosis and prognosis of the resultant speech deviance).
Brodnitz also explained that the frequently suggested utilization
of the residual tongue stump is dependent for success upon the

position, size and motility (if any) of the particular stump and its ability to make contact superiorly.

Among the vowels, he listed distortion of [i] and [e]. If the lip motility were absent or even reduced, [o] and [u] became indistinct. The semi vowels [w] and [hw] were similarly affected. The consonants [t] and [d], [s] and [z], [n], [θ] and [ð], and [ʃ] showed severe distortion. The [r] and [l] he reported as missing if the anterior part of the tongue had to be sacrificed. The intactness of the [k] and [g], and the [ŋ] were dependent on the motoric and tactile response of the posterior portion of the tongue.

For therapy, he suggested the use of a mirror to assist in substituting visual control for the disturbed motor and tactile feedbacks. Stretching and resistant exercises for the tongue residue as well as Froeschels pushing exercises were advocated. In speech compensation, the substitution of the lower lip against the upper teeth was again suggested for the lingua-dental phonemes. If the stump of the tongue can contact the palate, he stated an [l] can be formed. No suggestion was made concerning this sound if such contact is impossible. The [s] and [ʃ] may be lateralized or may be formed by blowing air through the teeth, also suggested in earlier papers. (No writer indicated a procedure where the patient is edentulous). A substitute for the lingual [r] can be found in the guttural (uvular) [r].

Four cases were reported as supporting the discussion. All four were described as partial rather than total excision. The first case of anchored tongue tip was treated for two months but the number of sessions was not specified. The speech was reported as almost normal. The second patient suffered a left lateral excision. He produced the lingua-dental sounds by use of the lip substitution and also achieved acceptable [s] and [l] and some improvement of the [k] and [g]. He discontinued treatment after four weeks and expressed satisfaction with his progress. Case three had to be discontinued after four weeks because of metastases which preceded the terminal stage; he had achieved the lip substitution for [t] and [d], and for [n]. The fourth patient was reported as very unintelligible, with [t] and [d], [s], and [r] missing, [l] severely distorted, [k] and [g] possible but indistinct, and the vowels all distorted.

Dr. Brodnitz mentioned drooling, dysphagia and depression as recurrent problems with glossectomy patients. He indicated the need for counseling. He suggested that the pushing exercises of Froeschel assist not only in the production of [k] and [g] phonemes but also in eliminating regurgitation and facilitating swallowing. He emphasized the part the speech clinician can play in reinforcing lip closure. Head, and consequently chin, elevation both help in control of drooling and in facilitation of active swallowing.

Massengill (1970) describes three glossectomy patients. He reports that the speech became increasingly distorted as larger percentages of the tongue were removed. The distortion did not appreciably interfere with communication. One patient was classed as total and two as partial glossectomees.

The Sixties and the Seventies

In 1968, "Total Glossectomy for Cancer," by Donaldson, appeared in the *American Journal of Surgery*. It reported the surgery procedures and survival rates for 14 patients with total excision of the tongue, chosen for the report from a population of 60. Included was an evaluation by the surgeon of the speech achieved, together with acknowledgment of the participation of the speech pathologist. The early unstructured experimental work with speech rehabilitation at the St. Louis Veterans Administration led to a planned pilot study, resulting in a paper titled "Compensatory Physiologic Phonetics for the Glossectomee," which was presented by Skelly in November, 1968, at the annual meeting of the American Speech and Hearing Association and in June, 1969, at the annual Head and Neck Cancer Conference at the University of Miami Medical School. Subsequently, it was published in February, 1971, in the *Journal of Speech and Hearing Disorders*. This paper reported a pilot study of 14 total and 11 partial glossectomees in an experimental approach to optimal compensatory movements. Pretherapy and posttherapy objective testing of intelligibility was carried out. Cinefluorographic examination of the successful speech compensations was analyzed. Consistent compensations were identified for all English glossal phonemes except the voiced and voiceless (th): [θ] and [ð]. Some specific techniques were perfected for developing the glossal phonemes. These proved effective with later cases. As hypothesized, considerable difference was revealed between the substitutions of the partial glossectomees and the compensations of those with total excision. Two further hypotheses evolved:

1. That swallow competence is a necessary antecedent of speech rehabilitation.
2. That there are phonatory components in glossectomee intelligibility improvement.

In November, 1969, a second paper, titled "Phonatory Aspects of Glossectomee Intelligibility," was presented by Skelly at the American Speech and Hearing Association annual meeting and repeated in June, 1970, at the Annual Head and Neck Cancer Conference at University of Miami Medical School. It is scheduled for publication in the *Journal of Speech and Hearing Disorders* in 1972. It reports a controlled therapy study involving 20 patients on the effects of specific vocal parameter manipulation on intelligibility improvement. Results indicated an optimal rate for these surgical patients differing from the normal. Pitch elevation, extention of pitch range and prolongation of vowels all appeared to be significantly related to improvement in communication.

In August, 1971, a third paper, "Glossectomee Speech Rehabilitation Procedures," from the same team was presented by Skelly at the International Congress of Logopedics and Phoniatrics at the University of Buenos Aires School of Medicine in Argentina. It provided directives for a detailed program of therapeutic techniques and procedures evolved from the prior research at the same clinic, reflecting clinical contact with over seventy glossectomee patients of varying involvement, excision, age and rehabilitation success. This will be published in June, 1972, by Ares of Argentina in the *Proceedings of the XV International Congress of Logopedics and Phoniatrics*.

PART TWO

EXPERIMENTATION

Chapter IV

COMPENSATORY PHYSIOLOGIC
PHONETICS

INTELLIGIBILITY

Two widely divergent views of the problem emerge from the literature of oral cancer and oral surgery. Many accept the idea that intelligibility is impossible when the tongue is completely removed. Some believe that intelligible speech develops after such surgery as a usual consequence of the passage of time and the exercise of some effort on the part of the patient. Possibly the optimistic attitude reflects the experience of those who have dealt with cases of partial excision, while a pessimistic view is taken by those who have attempted rehabilitation of patients with total loss of the tongue. The reporting team's clinical experience with 75 glossectomy patients to date tends to controvert both extreme views. Probably the critical distinction is the definition of "intelligibility."

In our 1969 survey of, and subsequent pilot therapy program with, 25 glossectomy patients, the speech of these patients on admission to the speech clinic program was not intelligible at a useful life-situation level. Untrained listeners unacquainted with the patient were not able to grasp his ideas in a conversation, even in an expected context. Trained listeners (the speech clinicians) had difficulty also. Success in communication by the patient was confined to a very limited vocabulary, which was understood only by that particular patient's immediate associates. Even here, listener comprehension was produced by numerous repetitions by the glossectomy speaker. Any achieved understanding was largely the result of an interested listener's developed ability to interpret the speaker's substitutions and distortions.

True intelligibility cannot be measured clinically in such limited terms. Such limited intelligibility cannot be described as being generally useful to the patient in diverse daily communication situations.

There is an apparent contradiction in the contrast of this initial assessment of the pilot group and the satisfactory level of articulation reflected in several of the studies previously reviewed. The divergence may be due to a number of factors. The research team was assessing patients with whom they were unfamiliar. They were judging the communication of these patients under the pressure of hospital interview situations with strange receptionist, clerks and other personnel. They were approaching the evaluations critically. They were comparing the patient's output to regional normal speech.

Possibly any person directly involved in the patient's treatment and consequently in his success loses at least some portion of his critical objectivity. Extensive knowledge of the patient's difficulties, gained over a period of therapeutic contact, tend to alter the criteria of success. The patient's output at any given assessment is compared not to a general standard or norm but to his output postoperatively.

Most of the studies reflecting a high level of intelligibility were based on only a very few subjects (2 to 5). The person reporting had some vested interest in the patient's success. Any listening audiences were presented with speech samples that were drilled prior to the presentation. The listeners were prepared to accept any intelligibility without a tongue as a rather remarkable achievement.

In our study of 25 glossectomees, 14 were totals and 11 were partials. All patients had biopsy-proved squamous cell carcinoma. Metastatic cancer of the cervical lymph nodes occurred in 13. Unilateral neck dissection was carried out in 16 and staged bilateral neck dissection in 7. The hyoid bone was removed in 6. The epiglottis was excised in 3, the soft palate altered in 3, and the gingiva altered in 1. Twenty-three were hemimandibulectomees and one was also a hemimaxillectomee. One was also a laryngectomee. Six of the total glossectomees had inadequate swallow, necessitating use of the Levin tube; otherwise, these patients aspirated liquid or food. The other total and all the partial glossec-

TABLE I

POSTOPERATIVE STATUS OF GLOSSECTOMY SUBJECTS
PARTIAL GLOSSECTOMEES

Clinician Ranking of Patient	Metastatic Cancer of Cervical Lymph Nodes	Unilateral Neck Dissection	Staged Bilateral Neck Dissection	Hyoid Bone Removed	Hemimandibu-lectomy	Epiglottis Removed	Soft Palate Altered	Levin Tube Feeding	Dysphagia	Laryngectomy	Hemimaxil-lectomy	Gingiva Altered
1					X							
2		X			X		X					X
3	X	X			X							
4					X							
5			X		X							
6					X							
7		X			X							
8	X	X			X							
9	X	X										
10	X	X										
11		X										

TABLE II

POSTOPERATIVE STATUS OF GLOSSECTOMY SUBJECTS
TOTAL GLOSSECTOMEES

Clinician Ranking of Patient	Metastatic Cancer of Cervical Lymph Nodes	Unilateral Neck Dissection	Staged Bilateral Neck Dissection	Hyoid Bone Removed	Hemimandibulectomy	Epiglottis Removed	Soft Palate Altered	Levin Tube Feeding	Dysphagia	Laryngectomy	Hemimaxillectomy	Gingiva Altered
1	X		X	L½	X							
2	X	X		X	X							
3		X		L½	X							
4			X		X	X						
5	X		X		X							
6		X		X	X							
7	X	X		X	X							
8			X		X					X		
9	X	X			X							
10	X		X					X	X			
11	X		X					X	X			
12	X						X	X	X			
13	X	X			X	X	X	X	X		X	
14	X	X			X							

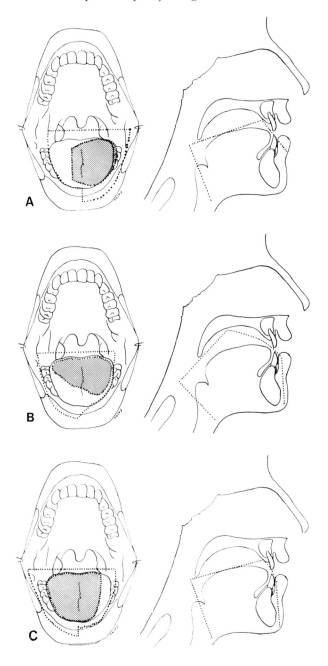

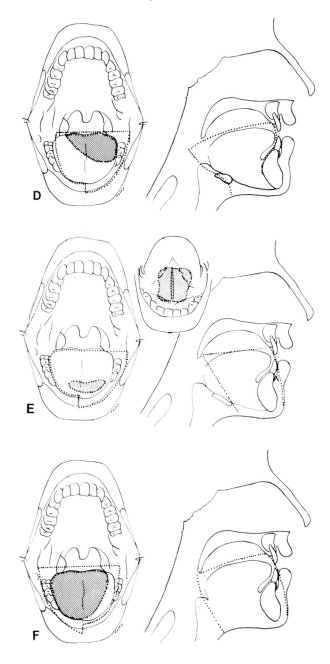

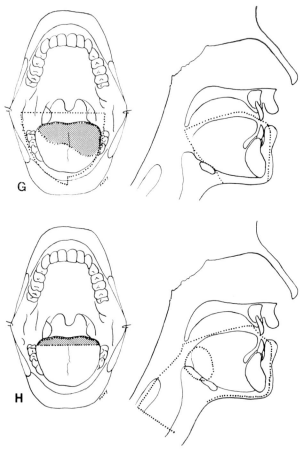

Figure 2 A–H. Schematic drawings of surgery of total glossectomees reported in Chapter IV as the first eight subjects.

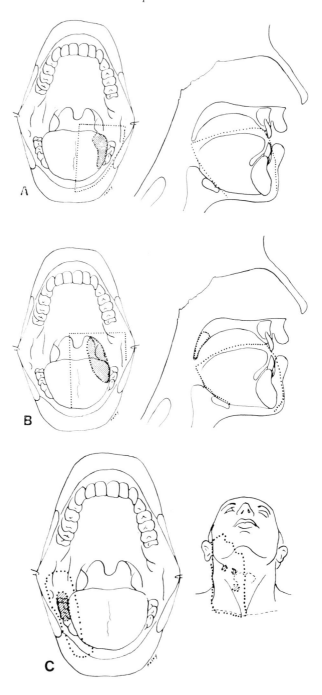

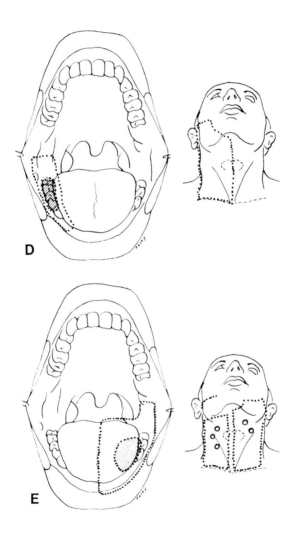

D

E

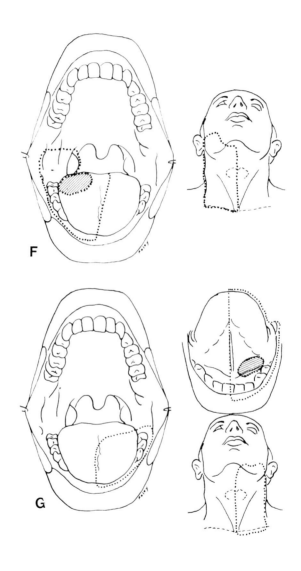

F

G

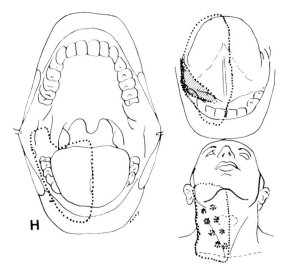

Figure 3 A–H. Schematic drawings of surgery of partial glossectomees reported in Chapter IV as first eight subjects.

tomees had swallowing ability sufficient to enable them to ingest foods and liquids without intubation.

Time lapse between surgery and admission to the speech program varied between nine months and nine years. Patients ranged in age from 44 to 71 years. One case of moderate bilateral hearing loss was discovered, with all other audiograms showing only mild losses. All patients involved in the program were able to travel to the hospital by public conveyance on an outpatient basis. Three of the partial glossectomy patients withdrew from the program at an early stage for various reasons.

ADMISSION TESTING

Patient intelligibility was assessed on admission to the program by means of the W-22 Phonetically Balanced Word Lists (1952) adapted by the Central Institute for the Deaf in St. Louis, under contracts with the Office of Naval Research and the Veterans Administration, from the Phonetically Balanced Word Lists of the Psycho-Acoustic Laboratory of Harvard University. This material was chosen because of its acoustic standardization for phonemic range and discrimination in the audiologic field.

In audiologic evaluation, the patient writes (or speaks) what he hears a test record saying. For the purpose of the glossectomy project, a transposed application was utilized.

The patient chose at random one of the eight arrangements of the list and recorded the words in stereo on an Ampex 600, twelve inches from the microphone, at three-second intervals at 40 dB amplification. Three untrained listeners, whose normal hearing had been verified, listened to the playback at the same level in free field in a clinic booth where ambient noise level seldom exceeds 20 dB, and wrote what they heard.

The three-man listening team for each patient was chosen from a pool of 27, so that any one listener was exposed to only three patients. The intent was to maintain listener-level stability, but avoid a list-learning factor. The average of the three listeners' scores was assigned as the patient's intelligibility score. Three staff clinicians ranked the patients clinically on intelligibility of their running speech. In the accompanying intelligibility test summaries, the patients are listed in the clinician-assigned order. There was complete agreement among the clinicians on the

TABLE III

INTELLIGIBILITY SUMMARY
TOTAL GLOSSECTOMEES

Clinician Ranking of Patients	CID W-22 PB *		Glossal * Monosyllables		Life Situation * Questions	
	Pre	Post	Pre	Post	Pre	Post
	%		%		%	
1	8	42	2	38	4	76
2	6	40	0	36	12	76
3	8	34	4	26	8	66
4	6	24	0	30	0	56
5	4	26	0	22	4	46
6	4	20	0	16	0	40
7	4	18	0	14	0	40
8 ***	0	18	0	12	0	26
9 **	0	0	0	0	0	0
10 **	0	0	0	0	0	0
11 **	0	0	0	0	0	0
12 **	0	0	0	0	0	0
13 **	0	0	0	0	0	0
14 **	0	0	0	0	0	0

* Perfect test score would be 100.
** Dysphagic.
*** Also laryngectomy.
Note: Rank order in which patients are listed was determined by consensus of three staff speech pathologists. The dysphagic patients (9 through 14) were all considered to rank 9th.

TABLE IV

INTELLIGIBILITY SUMMARY
PARTIAL GLOSSECTOMEES

Clinician Ranking of Patients	CID W-22 PB *		Glossal * Monosyllables		Life Situation * Questions	
	Pre	Post	Pre	Post	Pre	Post
	%		%		%	
1	16	46	10	30	56	86
2	24	42	20	50	56	88
3	12	36	16	30	42	76
4	20	40	20	40	54	78
5	12	34	20	34	40	65
6	12	34	16	26	40	60
7	8	26	14	24	40	58
8	6	24	10	20	36	56
9 **	6	—	12	—	24	—
10 **	8	—	10	—	28	—
11 **	6	—	10	—	26	—

* Perfect test score would be 100.
** Three patients dropped from program in the early stages.

order. Total glossectomees and partial glossectomees were ranked separately.

Because the CID W-22 PB lists include all the phonemes of English, and it may be that the major factor in glossectomee phonemic deviance lies in distortion of the glossal sounds only, the patients were similarly tested on devised lists of 50 monosyllables based on glossal consonant and vowel combinations. These monoglossal scores were compared with the PB scores. Difference and direction of difference were intended for utilization in individual therapy planning.

Since the basic aim of all intelligibility improvement is better communication for the patient's life situation, a functional test was devised for hospital use by the patient in actual communication situations. A list of 50 items of information was formulated, on which correct answers were independently available from hospital records of each patient. Questions on these, randomly arranged in segments of 25, were presented to patients by receptionists, clerks, secretaries, etc., who then recorded their understanding of the patient's replies. These were scored on successful transmission of information (see Appendix) .

Because of scant prior data on evaluation, treatment or progress of glossectomy patients, and especially because in this study preoperative recordings of the patient's speech were unavailable for progress comparisons, several types of assessment were deemed advisable. The PB scores were interpreted as indicating the patient's current intelligibility across all the phonemes of English. The glossal monosyllables indicated the deviance of each of the glossal sounds. The functional life-situation questions estimated the degree to which the phonemic deviance interfered with communication in an actual situation.

Much remains to be done in devising an adequate single test of intelligibility for these patients for use in admission, for therapy planning, as a measure of progress and hopefully, eventually as a prognostic instrument.

PILOT PROJECT

On the assumption that adequate compensations could be developed, could be consistent and could be useful in therapy, a clinical program was then undertaken. The exploratory therapeutic program included:

1. Exercises for improvement of excursion and control of the available articulators.
2. Drill for intelligibility of
   a. Vowels.
   b. Non-glossal consonants.
   c. Glossal consonants.
   d. Combinations of vowels with glossal consonants.
   e. Glossal consonants in ordinary context.
3. Systematic exploration of the available articulators for potential compensations for each glossal phoneme with each individual patient.
4. Application of any resulting useful compensatory patterns developed with one patient to therapy with the other patients.
5. Isolation of those compensations for each glossal phoneme most productive of intelligibility increase in any case.
6. Integration of these compensations in the therapeutic program with each patient under treatment.

After a 12-month project, the intelligibility assessments were repeated. Pretreatment and posttreatment scores are summarized in Tables III and IV.

CINEFLUOROGRAPHY PROCEDURES

Cinefluorographic studies for the purpose of identifying the physiologic compensations were then made of the five total glossectomees with highest rated intelligibility scores. The two partial glossectomees with highest scores in their group, as well as two normal speakers, were also filmed for comparison.

For the cinefluorography, the 16-mm camera recorded 24 frames /sec, using a Picker 8-in. 3000 brightness image intensifier. Shellburst linagraph film was used with magnetic sound recorded on a stereo Ampex 600 and dubbed to the shellburst. The filming was from $\frac{1}{2}$ to 5 ma pulsating x-ray, with the roentgen dosage to the subject of 2 rad, at a 24-in. distance from target to intensifier. Film development was by automatic processing. The films were examined for compensatory movement patterns on monosyllables from a glossal word list: gay, air, see, eel, rye, aisle, low, own, new, use; as well as the vowels [e], [aɪ], [o], [i], and [u].

Members of the team, working as a group, examined the cines in three runs of each subject, viewing on a 24-in. television monitor in the Radiology Service. This instrument produced exceptionally sharp, clear pictures. The films were next viewed projected on an auditorium-size film screen. This was followed with frame-by-frame viewing on a film analyzer by individual team members, repeated through several sessions, with attention focused in each session on a specific locus of compensation: lips, velum, uvula, cheeks, pharyngeal wall, epiglottis (where present), and mandible; as well as speed and synergies. Observations were exchanged and viewings on the analyzer repeated in group situation. No frame-by-frame measurements or superimpositions were achieved at this time, due to various limitations imposed on this pilot project. Team discussions following the multiple viewings resulted in consensus on observations reported.

INTELLIGIBILITY RESULTS

The six total glossectomee patients with inadequate swallow made no progress from their initial intelligibility assessment at zero score. Otherwise, differences were observed between total and partial glossectomees in both initial and terminal scores on all tests. The partial glossectomees achieved their gains in shorter time and fewer sessions. Some reached their plateau of progress in six months; all did within a year. Although the total glossectomees were assessed for the purposes of this pilot project at the end of the 12-month period, all were continued on the clinic schedule in hope of further progress, since plateaus were not reached at this time. If a patient makes no progress in any four weeks of treatment without explanatory circumstances, he is considered at plateau.

There was some bias inherent in the procedures and personnel utilized for the intelligibility scoring. Assessments were not all made by the same untrained listeners, as it was considered desirable to avoid a learning factor. However, this introduced individual listener and discrimination factors. Some control was achieved by carrying forward two thirds of any listener-group to the next listener-task each time. Thus, some constancy of group was maintained, yet the learning factor was minimized.

Independent assessments of intelligibility were made both pretreatment and posttreatment by three staff speech pathologists. Results at all levels were higher than scores of untrained listeners. The speech pathologists scored the upper half of each group 10 percent higher than untrained listeners and the lower half of each group 15 percent higher than untrained listeners. Aside from this differential, there was agreement in the ranking of the individual patients.

PARTIAL GLOSSECTOMEE ADAPTATIONS

Adaptive patterns of movement differed between the two groups, with the partial glossectomees making marked use of the residual tongue stump, rather than the more varied substitutions developed by the total glossectomy patients. It may be that the partial glossectomee can be treated as an articulation problem, since his adaptations appear to be modifications of the normal articulation patterns, as contrasted with the compensatory substitution movements of the total glossectomee.

There were some clinical indications that the type and extent of tongue section were related to speech clarity in the partial glossectomy group. Excision of the right or left half of the tongue appeared to require fewer speech adaptations than excisions including the entire tip. The flexibility of the residual tongue stump may also be a critical factor. The phonemes [z], [n] and [g] appeared to be produced by the partial glossectomee in a manner resembling the normal. If any flexible portion of the tongue remained, the partial glossectomee seemed able to approximate the phoneme [ð] and also [d] within acceptable phonemic limits. The most deviant sounds for these patients were [r] and [l].

TOTAL GLOSSECTOMEE COMPENSATIONS

In the total excision cases, among-patient consistency was observed in the achieved compensations. The team concluded that [z] was produced by means of a bilabial tension obstruction of the airstream, with the lips in much closer approximation than usual for this phoneme; [n] was produced by momentary velar contraction followed by a quick uvular relaxation, with the lips concurrently almost approaching true adduction; these patients appeared to differentiate [n] from [m] not only by degree of labial occlusion, but also by a shift in nasal resonance; [g] was produced by pharyngeal constriction, with slight bulging of the retroglossal pharyngeal wall, with the acoustic result resembling the German glottal; [d] was produced by utilizing the lower lip in contact with the upper teeth, or in the case of edentulous patients, with the upper alveolar ridge; [l] and [r] were produced by combination of pharyngeal, uvular and buccal movements, very similar in pattern for both sounds. For the [l], the uvula appeared to have some slight vibration which possibly provided the division of the airstream usually considered critical to the production of this phoneme. Some buccal constriction differences were also observed.

Both [ð] and [θ] remained problems for all the total glossectomees studied. One patient approximated this phoneme by an anterior thrust of the upper lip, passing it across the lower lip, terminating with explosion. This approach was not productive with any of the other patients.

Study of the films revealed compensatory movement for vowel production not previously observed clinically. The total glossectomy patients consistently utilized an anterior mandibular thrust at varying excursions on the vowels. This was not noted in the partial glossectomees or in normal subjects filmed.

LIMITATIONS

The work reported here has been only a beginning. Many limitations may be affecting any possible conclusions. Some of them are inherent in clinically based research, others hopefully will be controlled in subsequent studies. It may be well, however, to mention two such related factors. The speech intelligibility of these selected patients may be due largely to the particular surgical procedures in these cases, reported by Donaldson, Skelly and Paletta (1968). Some bias may have affected the project also because of the team's rehabilitation orientation.

FUTURE PROJECTS

Further studies now in progress or preparation seek to modify the limitations of the current report and hopefully will provide a base for more definitive conclusions. Preliminary spectrographic examination of glossectomy speech has been completed on the same patients. Since swallow competence appears to be related in these patients to development of speech intelligibility, a study of therapeutic approaches to dysphagia is underway.

SUMMARY

Compensatory articulation patterns on the glossal phonemes were developed clinically with the glossectomy patients through mandibular, labial, buccal and palatal adjustment and control. These were examined by cinefluorography. Compensatory patterns differed observably between total and partial glossectomees, with the latter making use of residual tongue stump in adaptive movements approximating the normal. The total glossectomees utilized truly compensatory patterns, with among-patient consistency in relation to developing intelligibility, as measured pretreatment and posttreatment.

A clinical population of 14 total and 11 partial glossectomees were examined. Three of the partial glossectomee patients withdrew at an early stage. Six of the total glossectomees made no progress. All six had dysphagia, with Levin tube feedings. The remaining 8 partial and 8 total glossectomees demonstrated no dysphagias. All made varying degrees of progress in intelligibility, as measured by CID W-22 PB work lists.

The partial glossectomees ranged between 6 per cent and 24 per cent intelligibility on admission and shifted to 24 per cent to 46 per cent intelligibility range after the therapy sequence. The total glossectomees ranged from 0 per cent to 8 per cent intelligibility on admission and shifted to 18 per cent to 42 per cent intelligibility range in the program.

Further studies in cinefluorography and acoustic spectrography, as well as dysphagia, seek to extend and improve the findings of this exploratory project.

Chapter V

DYSPHAGIA

RITA SOLOVITZ FUST

SWALLOWING

THE SWALLOWING function serves two distinct purposes. The first is the propulsion of food through the pharynx into the esophagus. The second is protection of the airway, both from above and below, from the entrance of food particles. Deglutition has been observed directly from individuals with facial defects, providing visualization of the movements of the oral and pharyngeal structures. It has been analyzed also by cinefluorography, cineradiography and electromyography.

An understanding of the basic physiology of swallowing is essential in understanding the dynamics of postsurgical deglutition and its handicapping effect on the glossectomy patient. The swallowing act is commonly described as a composite of three stages: oral, pharyngeal and esophageal. These three phases comprise a unified whole of intricately coordinated movements.

Oral Stage

During the oral stage of normal swallowing, the bolus of food is carried backward to the superior dorsum (midline) of the tongue. The position of the bolus between the tongue and palate is achieved by elevation of the tongue and depression of the soft palate. This conjunction of tongue and velum prevents the masticated mass from entering the pharyngeal airway (Weinberg, 1970). Furthermore, it effects propulsion of the bolus into the oropharynx. At this point, the hyoid bone and larynx are in maximally elevated positions. Fletcher (1970) describes the oral structures as forming a complete seal around the bolus: the lips and teeth anteriorly, the tongue and tensor-depressed soft palate

54

posteriorly, the hard palate superiorly, and the teeth and adjacent mucosa laterally.

The oral stage of swallowing is both a voluntary and reflexive activity. While it can be initiated voluntarily, it is normally a reflexive movement. Swallowing is initiated by stimulation of sensory receptors in the mouth. These receptors form a ring around the entrance to the oral pharynx and are found in the mucous membrane covering the anterior and posterior pillars of the fauces, the tonsils, soft palate, base of the tongue and the posterior pharyngeal wall. Hence, the swallow reflex may be initiated by stimulating the pharynx with a tongue blade.

Afferent pathways are mediated by sensory portions of the trigeminal nerve, the glossopharyngeal nerve and the pharyngeal plexus of the vagus. The oral movements of deglutition are effected by the anterior belly of the digastric, the mylohyoid and geniohyoid, which together carry the tongue and hyoid bone upward and forward. The geniohyoid and mylohyoid together form what is commonly termed the floor of the mouth. The stylohyoid muscle and posterior belly of the digastric draw the hyoid bone back and up. The mylohyoid and anterior belly digastricus are innervated by the trigeminal nerve (Cr.V), the geniohyoid is innervated by the hypoglossal nerve (Cr. XII) and the stylohyoid and posterior belly digastricus by the facial nerve (Cr. VII).

Pharyngeal Stage

The second or pharyngeal stage of swallowing is the transitional phase where peristaltic transport of the food bolus from mouth (oropharynx and hypopharynx) to the esophagus occur. The tongue releases the bolus as palate and tongue separate, effecting palatopharyngeal closure thus preventing food from entering the nasopharynx. The bolus of food is transported into the pharynx. The hyoid, tongue, pharynx, and larynx are all elevated at this time, the latter also being occluded to protect the airway. The airway is additionally protected by the horizontal position of the epiglottis as the tongue overrides the larynx. The cricopharyngeal sphincter relaxes, opening the esophagus for food entry. This phase of swallowing is primarily involuntary.

Many muscles are involved in this complex patterning of movement. The posterior belly of the digastric is contracted to elevate the larynx and to draw it under the base of the tongue for airway protection. The thyrohyoids likewise elevate the larynx. The palatopharyngeus and stylopharyngeus muscles raise the entire pharynx. Contraction of the tensor velipalatine and intrinsic muscles of the tongue move the mouth and oropharynx upward. Innervation of these muscles is provided by the hypoglossal (Cr. XII) and glossopharyngeal (Cr. IX) nerves.

Esophageal Stage

The primary event of the third or esophageal stage of swallowing is the entry of the bolus into the lumen of the esophagus. Reflexive peristalsis of the pharyngeal and esophageal muscles precedes the opening of the P-E segment. During this phase, the closure mechanism of the larynx is active to prevent airway penetration. The tongue and pharyngeal muscles are also contracted. Subsequent to this action, the larynx descends again and is opened. Layers of smooth muscle within the esophagus carry on peristaltic transport of the food into the stomach. The tongue, palate and hyoid then return to their pre-swallow positions.

During the esophageal stage, the posterior belly digastric and stylohyoid muscles elevate and retract the hyoid bone and base of the tongue. Contraction of the esophageal sphincter is effected by combined action of the laryngopharyngeus muscles, the inferior pharyngeal constrictors and the esophageal muscles. Innervation is provided by the vagus (Cr. X) nerve.

Most recent studies of frequency of swallowing reveal that human beings swallow approximately 590 times daily—146 times while eating, 394 times while awake but not eating, and 50 times during sleep (Subtelny, 1965). Averages for volumes of water consumed per swallow were reported by Jones and Work (Fletcher, 1970) as follows: 21.3 cc per swallow by men, 13.6 cc per swallow by women, and 4.6 cc per swallow by $1\frac{1}{4}$– to $3\frac{1}{2}$–year–old children.

POSTOPERATIVE DYSPHAGIA

An interruption in the normal functioning of the swallowing mechanism is a common postoperative problem for the glossectomy patient. While this form of dysphagia is physically based, there may be considerable psychological or emotional overlay. Dysphagia is a residual of the surgical procedure which included severance of several muscles involved in the swallowing process. Postoperative absence of the tongue or portion of the tongue with its intrinsic and extrinsic muscles is the most obvious factor contributing to the postsurgical dysphagia, although the anterior and posterior bellies of the digastric and the stylohyoid are usually removed as well. If a floor-of-the-mouth resection is performed, the mylohyoid and geniohyoid muscles are resected. While impaired deglutition may follow limited surgical procedures such as thyroid lobectomy or radical neck dissection, true dysphagia results from larger resections of the tongue, larynx and pharynx (Trible, 1967). Finally, injury to the internal branch of the superior laryngeal nerve, which provides sensory fibers to the pharynx, can stifle pharyngeal sensation. Stimulation of the pharyngeal area triggers the involuntary swallowing movements of the tongue, soft palate and pharynx.

ROLE OF SPEECH PATHOLOGIST

The patient with defective functioning of the speech mechanism following head and neck surgery should be referred routinely to the speech pathologist for a speech evaluation (including assessment of vocal functioning) and possible speech and voice rehabilitation. Such a patient usually presents a dysphagic condition in addition to his communicative problem. If recovery of this function has not occurred spontaneously in the early postoperative period due to extent of surgery, postsurgical complication or psychological factors, it will be of primary concern to the speech pathologist. It is on the mechanism serving the vegetative, animalistic oral functions of chewing, sucking and swallowing that human speech depends. Many of the same oral structures are involved in speaking and swallowing, creating an anatomical overlay, if not a functional or physiological one.

The patient's recovery of normal functioning of swallowing comes within the realm of total patient care. The dysphagic patient is in danger of aspirating liquids or solid foods which inadvertently enter the airway in his attempts to swallow. This problem may require the use of a suctioning machine or even emergency tracheotomy procedures in extreme cases. While many persons on the rehabilitation team may be quite validly involved with the patient's inability to swallow, it is properly the responsibility of the surgeon to deal with it.

However, the speech pathologist may be called upon to assist the physician in treating the patient's swallowing problem. The dynamics of deglutition, normal and nonfunctional, as well as therapeutic techniques for retraining the swallow should be of interest and distinct value to the speech pathologist.

The role of the speech pathologist as "myofunctional therapist" (Garliner, 1966) has been questioned. Several authors have challenged the position of the speech pathologist in conducting such therapeutic exercise. Shelton (1963) contended that the speech specialist should deal with impaired muscles only insofar as the problem precludes or interferes with speech learning. He should, however, work cooperatively with the physiatrist on proper and common skills. More fundamental functions of management of saliva and swallowing should be dealt with prior to, or concomitant with, any remedial speech program. Herberman (1958) reported that as swallowing skills and salivary continence improved in patients receiving therapy to facilitate swallowing, concomitant changes were observed in articulation and speech intelligibility.

When a patient who is not swallowing is referred for speech rehabilitation, the physician's attention should be directed to the patient's need for this treatment. In such cases, the speech pathologist may be the person most suited for working with the dysphagia. Such factors as the speech pathologist's greater availability for intensive work with the patient, understanding of and patience with the communication problem, rapport with the patient, and detailed knowledge of the oropharyngeal structure and function may render him best suited for the task. In all such instances, he must work in close cooperation with the physician. When medical assistance is not immediately available, techniques should be limited to those involving the "dry" swallow (without liquid or food) to eliminate any danger of aspiration.

Following surgery, patients are fed through a nasogastric tube inserted 48 hours postoperatively. Most physicians report that the nasogastric tube may be removed as early as 21 days after surgery. This period may be as much as 6 or 8 weeks, depending on the nature of the surgery and any postoperative complications, as well as the motivation of the patient. The surgeon will then encourage the patient to attempt swallowing. Many patients spontaneously recover the ability to swallow and need little in the way of therapeutic aid.

Rehabilitative measures usually begin with the patient's diet. The patient is encouraged to begin swallowing liquids or soft, "mushy" foods. Where the patient's tongue is partially or completely absent, liquids may be easiest to take because they can be directed to the oropharynx, bypassing the need for lingual movement. Indeed, many patients, during initial stages of swallowing recovery, will compensate for lack of tongue movement by tilting back the head, encouraging the liquid to run back to the pharynx by gravitational pull. Donaldson *et al.* (1968) reported an alternative method to the normal pharyngeal swallow where patients have lost their pharyngeal reflex. These patients learn to relax the cricopharyngeus muscle voluntarily and pour liquids into the esophagus without need of pharyngeal constrictor movement. Some physicians feel that liquids, particularly water, are difficult to control due to lack of texture. Hence, semiliquid or soft foods may be the more effective initial agents for redevelopment of swallowing.

Various devices can be used for implementing food intake. Herberman (1958) reported the use of a small plastic plunger-type pastry tube which is filled with diluted baby food. The device is inserted into the faucal area of the mouth, where the food is released. By holding his breath, the patient elevates his soft palate, closing off the nasal passage to prevent nasal regurgitation. Another implement is the long-handled spoon used to deposit food in the faucal area. The kitchen blender is useful in preparing foods of the appropriate consistency.

The literature of surgery and physical medicine has little to offer to date on specific techniques for retraining swallowing. Perhaps because many areas of head and neck surgery are relatively new, particularly supraglottic and hemilaryngectomy procedures, the focus of attention remains at present on the surgical procedures themselves. Specific postoperative therapeutic techniques are based largely on knowledge of anatomy and physiology, clinical observation, and trial and error, passed on from physician to physician.

Before attempting to work with the dysphagic postoperative patient, the clinician must understand fully the nature and extent

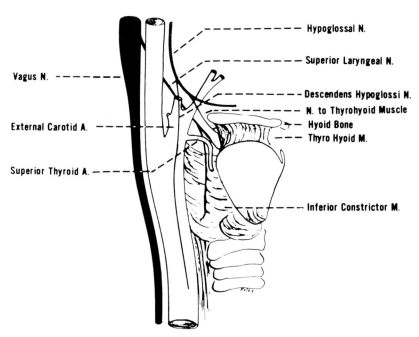

Figure 4. Diagram showing the approximate relative locations of the superior laryngeal nerve, its internal and external branches, the nerve to the thyrohyoid muscle, and the hyoid bone. The importance of the branches of the superior laryngeal nerve to the act of swallowing is discussed in the text.

of the disorder. The surgical report will reveal which nerves and muscles have been sacrificed and which are preserved. The patient's postoperative progress is also relevant. Whether he is adapting to his swallowing deficit, such as swallowing liquids with effort, will determine at what point therapeutic treatment should begin.

Initially the clinician must observe the patient's attempt to swallow. He can feel the movement or lack of movement of the thyroid cartilage which normally rises and lowers. The gag reflex can be visualized upon stimulation of the posterior pharyngeal wall with a tongue blade or cotton swab. Observations of palatal movement and mobility of any tongue stump are pertinent.

REHABILITATION TECHNIQUES

Imagery is an effective technique in retraining the swallow. The clinician initially may convey the image to the patient by encouraging him to "swallow hard." Visual cues may aid. Image building may be achieved by description in laymen's terms of the swallowing function or use of diagrams to depict the various structures and movements. Wherever feasible, the clinician should demonstrate an exercise before asking the patient to attempt it.

Tactile sensation and kinesthetic awareness of positions and relationships of oral structures may be utilized successfully. The clinician may have the patient touch the clinician's neck in the area of the thyroid cartilage to feel its normal upward, then downward, movement during swallowing. Simple chewing, blowing, puckering or sucking (through a straw) exercises can develop or increase the patient's awareness of his lips, tongue and cheeks and the various movements they perform. These procedures by no means suggest that these movements involve the same muscles or movements as in swallowing. However, various functional oral movements can help develop awareness, feeling and control of the oral structures.

Pushing exercises are an extremely valuable technique for re-training the swallow. They were first introduced by Froeschels (Froeschels *et al.,* 1955) for patients with paralysis of the soft palate. Weiss (in Froeschels) reported their application to patients with recurrent nerve paralysis (abductor and adductor paralysis of the vocal cords), and Kastein (also in Froeschels) used them with neurological problems affecting the functions of phonation, respiration and glutination.

Pushing exercises are based on the rationale that sudden voluntary contraction of a group of muscles causes concomitant contraction of other muscle groups, reinforcing the function of the first group. Brodnitz (1965), who recommended pushing exercises in treating hypofunctional voice cases, brought this principle to bear on reciprocal contraction of the laryngeal sphincter (vocal fold closure) and contraction of the muscles of the shoulders during heavy lifting, pushing or pulling. Hence, when the shoulder muscles are exerted, there occurs also immobilization of the thoracic cavity in an expiratory position and firm closure of the glottis.

Froeschels *et al.* (1955) reported the use of pushing exercises with patients having neural impairments of the glossopharyngeal, vagus and mandibular division of the trigeminal nerve. Damage to these nerves resulted in inactivity or reduced activity of the soft palate and therefore difficulty with swallowing. Pushing exercises, then, stimulate contraction of both the laryngeal sphincter and the velum, which are similarly mobile during normal swallowing.

The pushing exercises consist of simultaneous movement (straining) of the arms with phonation—or for swallowing therapy, with the swallow. The clinician may begin by having the patient push while phonating "ah," the means of effecting glottic closure for phonation in voice therapy. The most effective pushing technique for inducing the swallow is actually a modification of the Froeschels method used by Kastein in treating patients with breathing and swallowing difficulties. In this application, the patient is seated in a chair with his hands clutching the edges of the chair at his sides, palms downward. He is told to push against the seat of the chair, raising himself up from the seat as he phonates "ah." As the patient pushes and phonates, his attention should be called to the feeling of moderate tension in the back of the mouth and throat. Awareness of muscular contraction can be reinforced by having the patient close his eyes and repeat the act, envisioning it in imagination. Other vowel sounds may be used alternately.

Once this procedure has been established, the patient is told to swallow as he pushes, envisioning and feeling the same pharyngeal (velar) and laryngeal contraction. Constant repetition of this exercise is needed for the patient to recreate the coordinated pattern of movements in swallowing and so eventually stabilize the sequence.

The patient is instructed to practice five to ten pushes with swallowing every half hour in his hospital room for the first few days. During that time, he may alternate phonation with swallowing for each pushing act to reinforce velar and laryngeal contraction and to provide some task variety. Frequency of practice may be reduced to five to ten times every hour on the third day and less thereafter, depending on progress. The patient should work with the clinician two sessions each day, each of which should be terminated well before the patient experiences fatigue. Frequency of these sessions can be reduced as the patient progresses.

As consistency and ease of swallowing develop, the physical push may be gradually eliminated. The patient is told to alternate a push and swallow movement using merely the remembrance (image, imagination) of pushing as he swallows. The clinician's goal is such vivid carryover of the visual and kinesthetic image of pushing that the actual pushing exercise is faded out completely.

The patient can attempt swallowing liquids or soft foods, whichever are easier for him, on the ward. The pushing image principle must be utilized. The patient may find that swallowing actual food is easier than the dry swallow, as it may stimulate more reflexive movement of the swallowing mechanism. The actual pushing exercise may be inserted as needed when the patient is first attempting blended foods, but he should be relying more and more on the utilization of imagery to achieve the desired effect.

The pushing effect can also be achieved by pulling actions. The patient can pull up on the chair seat or clasp his hands in front of his chest with arms horizontal and pull in opposite directions. Another method is holding onto and pulling oneself forward on a sheet or towel tied to the foot of the bed, suggested for bedridden patients.

COUNSELING

As with any rehabilitative endeavor, the person dealing with the dysphagic patient must be sensitive to the patient's psychological status. From a cosmetic standpoint, head and neck surgery, particularly if it is more extensive than excision of the tongue, may result in considerable disfigurement of the patient. The person who has undergone a partial mandibulectomy is one example. Without a complete mandible, this individual presents a characteristic "Andy Gump," somewhat chinless, appearance. This not only handicaps his swallowing and management of saliva with the consequent socially embarrassing drooling but is cosmetically deforming. His physical appearance may be only temporary, for the reconstructive phase of his rehabilitation may include surgical insertion of a "false" mandible to replace the resected bone and return the patient's mandible to a more normal contour. Various synthetic materials have been utilized for this purpose, including vitallium or silicone rubber. One of the newest procedural advances in surgical reconstruction is insertion of a mandibular prosthesis made of siliconized rubber and Kirchner wires at the time of the surgical resection. This procedure enables immediate restoration of mandibular function and appearance (McQuarrie, 1971).

The surgeon is often faced with the patient who *will not* swallow or *thinks* he cannot swallow, as opposed to one who actually cannot. Trible (1967) offers the opinion that a high incidence of concurrent alcoholism on the part of the patient increases the problem. Certainly such behavior may be related to a wide range of psychological traits, intelligence factors, education and socioeconomic level of the individual. All patients should be preoperatively prepared to expect a temporary inability to swallow as a postoperative residual. They may be reassured by knowing that many glossectomees have regained the swallowing function. Without such advance information, the speechless dysphagic patient regaining consciousness may experience severe emotional trauma. Believing his difficulty to be unique, he may falsely conclude that his surgery was unsuccessful and even that he is dying. This topic should be included also in the postoperative counseling of the family.

Chapter VI

PHONATORY ASPECTS OF
GLOSSECTOMEE INTELLIGIBILITY

D URING A 12-month period extending from July, 1967, through June, 1968, 25 glossectomized patients were examined by the speech pathology staff at the Veteran's Administration Hospital Audiology and Speech Pathology Service. The speech of these patients was characterized by extreme articulatory and phonological distortions. The voices were found to have an extremely low pitch and a very narrow pitch range. A common gutteral quality, confounded by excessive pharyngeal and oral noise, compounded the intelligibility problem.

A clinical project was undertaken to explore the effect of vocal parameter manipulation on certain aspects of the intelligibility of glossectomees, i.e. low frequencies, guttural quality and extraneous noise.

Sixty-eight cases were available from clinic records. Of these, 43 had already had varying amounts of compensatory articulation therapy, as previously reported (Skelly, Spector, Donaldson, Brodeur and Paletta 1971a).

These treated patients were retested for their individual current intelligibility scores using the Every Day Speech Sentences, Lists E and I (Davis and Silverman, 1970). These sentences were constructed so that in each 10 sentences, 50 critical words occur for the scoring of intelligibility. The same twenty sentences were recorded in a different order by each patient on a 600 Ampex tape recorder at 40 dB in a sound-treated room. Under the same conditions, each was scored by three clinicians unfamiliar with the patient or the material. Ten judges participated, each judging the tapes of three patients. (Interjudge reliability was previously established in a pilot intelligibility study with dysarthrics in which these judges were in 92% agreement on articulation scoring of the 50 test items on 25 patients). The average of the three scores for each patient was considered his preproject intelligibility score.

Each patient also recorded a series of seven words involving seven phonemes usually classified as glossal: [ð], [z], [d], [l], [n], [r], [g]. Three trials on each word were recorded for each patient. All word samples were examined by spectrography for consistency on repetition, vowel duration, noise, formants and harmonic range. Also, three staff clinicians who had been involved in the patient's prior compensatory articulation therapy ranked the patient's intelligibility from interview judgments.

The initial test scores fell into five deciles. For the therapy project, ten patients were chosen by selecting two randomly from each decile. In two cases, a second choice was made because the patient first selected was not available for the required experimental period. A control group of ten cases was similarly chosen, but received no therapy during this period.

All patients have had biopsy-proved squamous cell carcinoma. In the experimental group, five had metastatic cancer of the cervical lymph nodes, five had unilateral neck dissection, five had staged bilateral neck dissection, six had alteration of the hyoid bone. Nine were hemimandibulectomies and one had the epiglottis removed (see Table V).

In the control group, four had metastatic cancer of the lymph nodes, eight had unilateral neck dissection, and two had staged bilateral neck dissection. Ten were hemimandibulectomies, one with soft palate alteration and one with gingival alteration (see Table VI).

Time lapse between surgery and admission to the speech program varied between 16 weeks and 9 years. Patients ranged in age from 39 to 72 years of age. All had swallowing ability sufficient to enable them to ingest foods and liquids without intubation. All were able to travel to the hospital by public or personal conveyance on an outpatient basis. All had at least four months of compensatory articulation therapy, during which measurable improvement had occurred, although none had yet achieved successful production of [ð].

TABLE V

POSTOPERATIVE STATUS OF GLOSSECTOMEE EXPERIMENTAL SUBJECTS

Clinician Ranking of Patient	Metastatic Cancer of Cervical Lymph Nodes	Unilateral Neck Dissection	Staged Bilateral Neck Dissection	Hyoid Bone Removed	Hemimandibulectomy	Epiglottis Removed	Soft Palate Altered	Gingiva Altered	Edentulous
1	X	—	X	L1½	X	—	—	—	—
2	X	X	—	X	X	—	—	—	X
3	—	X	—	L1½	X	—	—	—	X
4	—	—	X	—	—	X	—	—	X
5	—	X	—	X	X	—	—	—	X
6	X	X	—	—	X	—	—	—	X
7	X	X	X	X	X	—	—	—	X
8	—	—	—	—	X	—	—	—	X
9	—	X	X	X	X	—	—	—	X
10	X	—	X	—	X	—	—	—	X

TABLE VI

POSTOPERATIVE STATUS OF GLOSSECTOMEE CONTROL GROUP

Clinician Ranking of Patient	Metastatic Cancer of Cervical Lymph Nodes	Unilateral Neck Dissection	Staged Bilateral Neck Dissection	Hyoid Bone Removed	Hemimandib-ulectomy	Epiglottis Removed	Soft Palate Altered	Gingiva Altered	Edentulous
1	—	X	—	—	X	—	—	—	—
2	—	X	—	—	X	—	X	—	X
3	X	—	—	—	X	—	—	X	X
4	—	X	X	—	X	—	—	—	X
5	—	X	X	—	X	—	—	—	X
6	—	X	—	—	X	—	—	—	X
7	—	X	—	—	X	—	—	—	X
8	X	X	—	—	X	—	—	—	X
9	X	X	—	—	X	—	—	—	X
10	X	X	—	—	X	—	—	—	X

TABLE VII
FREQUENCY AND DURATION MEASURES OF SEVEN GLOSSAL MONOSYLLABLES EXPERIMENTAL GROUP

Pretherapy and Posttherapy

Clinician Ranking	red *K Hz hi	red dur.**	dough K Hz hi	dough dur.	so K Hz hi	so dur.	no K Hz hi	no dur.	go K Hz hi	go dur.	low K Hz hi	low dur.	row K Hz hi	row dur.
1. Pre	6.0	.72	3.0	.80	3.0	.68	3.0	.76	3.0	.60	3.0	.76	3.0	.72
Post	6.5	.56	5.5	.56	5.5	.48	5.0	.64	7.5	.52	6.0	.64	7.0	.52
2. Pre	4.0	.66	2.5	.52	3.5	.56	2.5	.66	2.5	.52	2.5	.56	2.5	.66
Post	4.5	.58	5.0	.48	5.0	.52	5.5	.66	5.0	.46	5.5	.54	4.5	.54
3. Pre	3.5	.88	3.0	.68	3.0	.56	3.0	.88	2.0	.56	3.0	.68	3.0	.88
Post	4.0	.68	5.0	.52	7.0	.52	4.0	.72	4.0	.48	4.5	.54	4.0	.56
4. Pre	3.0	.84	2.5	.76	3.0	.66	1.5	.96	3.0	.66	1.5	.76	2.5	.96
Post	3.5	.74	6.0	.76	4.0	.64	5.0	.80	4.5	.64	4.0	.64	3.5	.58
5. Pre	3.0	.94	1.5	.76	3.0	.66	1.0	.80	3.0	.66	1.0	.76	1.5	.80
Post	3.5	.74	3.0	.70	3.5	.66	3.0	.80	3.5	.62	3.0	.68	3.5	.60
6. Pre	2.5	1.05	2.5	1.04	2.5	.80	2.5	1.12	2.5	.80	2.5	.76	2.5	.94
Post	3.5	.96	3.5	.96	3.0	.68	3.0	1.04	3.0	.68	3.0	.52	3.0	.64
7. Pre	2.0	1.19	1.0	.84	1.5	.76	1.5	.76	1.5	.76	1.5	.76	1.0	.84
Post	2.5	1.09	2.5	.72	2.5	.52	1.5	.64	2.5	.56	3.0	.64	2.0	.80
8. Pre	.5	.29	.5	.21	.5	.27	.5	.29	.5	.27	.5	.27	.5	.29
Post	2.0	.29	1.0	.21	1.5	.27	2.0	.29	1.0	.27	1.5	.27	1.0	.29
9. Pre	.5	.20	.5	.20	.5	.20	.5	.20	.5	.20	.5	.20	.5	.20
Post	.5	.25	.5	.25	.5	.25	.5	.25	.5	.25	.5	.25	.5	.25
10. Pre	.5	.25	.5	.25	.5	.25	.5	.25	.5	.25	.5	.25	.5	.25
Post	.5	.25	.5	.25	.5	.25	.5	.25	.5	.25	.5	.25	.5	.25
Normal Controls	8.0	.460	5.5	.420	8.0	.480	5.5	.560	7.5	.480	8.0	.520	7.5	.48

* Harmonic frequency high in thousands (K).
** Duration in seconds.

A therapeutic program was designed and carried out over a four-month period, with weekly sessions and assigned home drills. Selected monthly sentence tests and word sonagrams were used to check techniques and progress.

At the termination of the project, patients were retested on the same materials as on admission. These were scored in the same fashion by the same judges, with one replacement. Glossal word sonagrams were again printed. Duration and high-frequency measures were determined for the words "red," "dough," "zoe," "no," "go," "low," "row." None of the group achieved an acceptable production of the word "though."

Duration and frequency high were measured on the sonagram print in millimeters against the horizontal time scale by which 1 mm equaled .08 sec. The vertical scale located the high harmonics in C's up to 8 KHz against the sonagram print of a 5 CHz pure tone (see Table VII).

Means of duration and high frequency for the seven test words on four male normal speakers yielded .490 duration mean and 8000 Hz characteristic high frequency.

THERAPY GOALS AND METHODS

Therapeutic goals were established as
1. Reduction of oral and pharyngeal noise.
2. Appropriate adjustment of vowel duration.
3. Elevation of habitual pitch.
4. Extension of total pitch range.
5. Improvement of resonance for higher harmonics.

The sound-chewing exercises described by Brodnitz (1965) were considered applicable to all four therapy goals, particularly in noise reduction on phonation and elevation of habitual low pitch. The vowel prolongation drills used by actors were directed toward rate and resonance shift. Improved control of air emission was attempted by arresting expiration, building up pressure, then phonating. The vowels were produced first for maximum duration, then for maximum energy in minimum duration. Exercise for short, intense, reliable repetition of vowels was emphasized for the glossectomees early in therapy. The maximum-duration drills were introduced later in the program.

Reduction in undesirable pharyngeal noise was sought through a sequence of several steps. A wide, relaxed yawn initiated the series. Vowel phonation followed, accompanied by a manual pull upward on the chair seat. Sound chewing preceded exercises for control of phonation, duration and articulatory movement. Drills for oral size and shape alteration terminated in the yawned vowel. The patient then attempted an upward arpeggio after a second yawn. When any pitch shift was achieved, immediate repetition was encouraged, with the aim of stabilizing the pitch shift and increasing the vowel duration. Daily best-scores monitored by stopwatch provided some incentive.

Boone's (1971) excellent chapter on problems of resonance had much relevant information for therapy planning. He comments on the high pitch levels characteristic of strident voice. Since the glossectomee's characteristic low pitch and guttural quality may be reinforced by a pharyngeal cul-de-sac type of resonance which may be the extreme opposite of the strident voice, deliberate exercises for stridency were utilized to promote desirable pitch elevation for the glossectomee.

When warranted by success with the vowels, the same approaches were next applied to words from the non-glossal word lists, then to the glossal word lists in ascending order of difficulty and finally to phrases and sentences (see Appendix). Pauses for meaning were utilized. Word emphasis for meaning was included in the drill. Pitch pattern variation for meaning was attempted. An imagery approach was of considerable value in pitch elevation.

I go DOWN the mine.
I go UP the tower—up—up—up.
A boy is SHORT.
A man is TALL—tall—tall—tall.
The valley is LOW.
The mountain is HIGH—hi—hi—hi.
Father said NO.
Mother said YES—yes—yes—yes.

The customary inflectional patterns of English provided some profitable drill also. Short simple questions were utilized to elicit the usual rising inflection. When successful, this was combined with the high imagery concept.

Example: Going up?   Is he tall?   Is it very high?

Two problems arose in parameter manipulation. Usually in acoustics, the faster the rate, the higher the pitch. Also, the higher the intensity, the higher the pitch. In both instances, the converse is also true. Reduction in intensity is frequently utilized in therapy to lower undesirably high pitch. In the glossectomy therapy, it was desirable to slow the rate but elevate the pitch. It was also considered advantageous to diminish the intensity as an aid to noise reduction but at the same time avoid lowering the pitch.

A limited-purpose therapy was utilized on a series of short drill sentences. The objective was to record the sentence accomplishing the primary goal of pitch control regardless of rate, then repeat, maintaining the pitch but reducing the rate. On the following trial, the aim was to achieve the pitch control at high intensity, then repeat, sustaining pitch but reducing intensity. The final unit varied and combined all three. This appeared to be the most difficult subgoal in the project in measure of time and effort but was very profitable in terms of weekly score increase.

There are a number of additional considerations in any design of pitch therapy. Some of these were involved in the glossectomee program. None of the subjects displayed any emotional maladjustment affecting the therapy. Two subjects required auditory discrimination drills. One displayed some apparent deficit in tonal memory which may be highly relevant to his final low score. All had common problems in hypertension at initiation of the program and varying individual difficulties in some motor synergies. The auditory discrimination drills were regarded as legitimate aspects of voice improvement. No specific treatment was provided otherwise in these areas.

SONOGRAPHIC ASPECTS OF GLOSSECTOMEE INTELLIGIBILITY

In this project, highly observable differences were noted between a glossectomee sonagram and the normal printout in all cases on inspection of the admission sonagrams of the glossal word list. The least intelligible speaker had the least consistency on repetition; the most intelligible speaker had the greatest consistency. He was as stable as the normal controls.

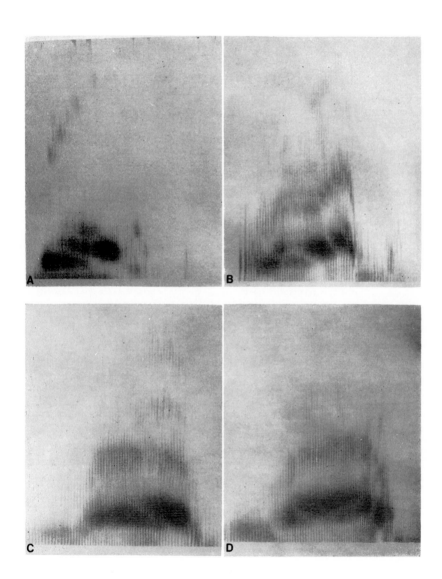

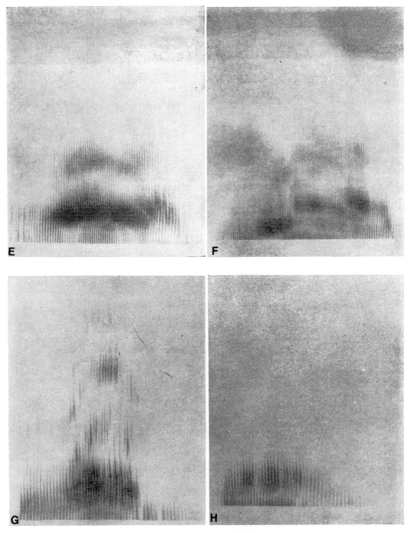

Figure 5 A–H. Sample sonagrams of eight patients speaking the same monosyllable, arranged in order of intelligibility.

The glossectomees displayed a tendency to diverge in duration from the time base of the normal speaker. Those with a shorter duration than the normal speaker were among the least intelligible. The more intelligible had duration spans beyond the normal, with the degree of difference consistently related to the intelligibil-

ity rank. Although the glossectomee speaker with highest intelligibility score had the least deviance, his duration was approximately 50 per cent longer than the normal. The cut-off point for
useful intelligibility occurred at about three times the normal
duration.

The first formant frequency band appeared to extend over a
wider range for the less intelligible and to decrease in range consistently as intelligibility improved. This and the characteristic
low pitch of the subjects were consistent with the formant studies
by House (1960). "Increasing the formant band widths of the
synthetic vowels resulted in a systematic drop in the level of all
formants. The formants in 'natural' speech are narrow rather than
wide (when *narrow* and *wide* are terms descriptive of two sets
of band-width measures in the speech literature)." The less intelligible speakers displayed in the first formant a greater concentration of energy than usual in comparison with the second
formant.

The second formant was absent in the unintelligible speaker's
sonagrams. It appeared weak and ill-defined in the less intelligible.

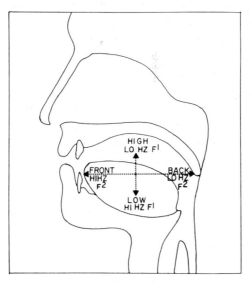

Figure 6. Vowel formant relationships to tongue position in the normal
mouth.

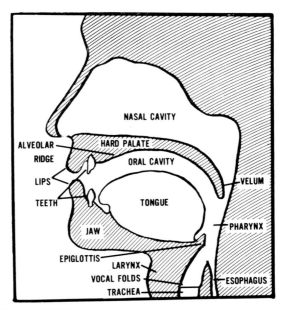

Figure 7A. Normal articulator and resonator balance.

It became more strongly defined and showed greater energy concentration in comparison with the first formant as intelligibility increased. This was consistent with the intelligibility study by Thomas (1968). "Clipped speech which contains only second formant information is highly intelligible (71.1%), while that containing only first formant information is virtually unintelligible (7.6%)."

In all the clinical spectrograms of unintelligible and least intelligible speakers, a widely distributed random noise pattern appeared and showed highest intensity at the lower frequencies. Consistently, the lower the intelligibility score, the narrower the speaker's frequency range and the more limited the harmonic range.

Since the first formant is not prime in intelligibility, while the second formant is (Thomas, 1968), compensatory vertical adjustment (F_1) was less important than compensatory horizontal adjustment (F_2) (see Fig. 6). Cinefluorographic examination indicated the glossectomee probably achieved the latter by anterior mandibular thrust (Skelly *et al.*, 1971a). The same study indicated some

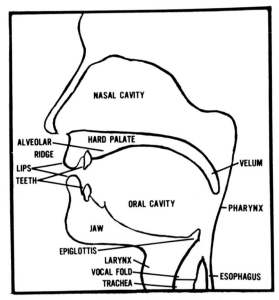

Figure 7. B, Excision of the tongue produces an extreme imbalance of the resonator couplings. Compare size and shape of oral and nasal chambers in A with those in B.

compensation for the vertical axis by labial adjustments. When shape of the vocal tract changes, differences will be noted in the formant frequencies, which may not coincide with those of the harmonics (Hoops, 1969). In the glossectomy patient, surgery has considerably altered the vocal tract tube, often in a highly individual configuration.

Coupling the nasal cavity creates a basically different vocal tract shape in normal speakers. In the glossectomee, the new size of the oral cavity often produces an extreme imbalance in the coupling (see Fig. 7). From both this imbalance and possible reduction of velar competence as a necessary consequence of the surgery, extreme antiresonances may result, which suppress parts of the speech spectrum. With the absence of the tongue in the glossectomee, the size and shape of the oral cavity are changed. Its ratio to the nasal and pharyngeal resonators is also necessarily altered (see Fig. 8). Problems in resonance adjustment occur.

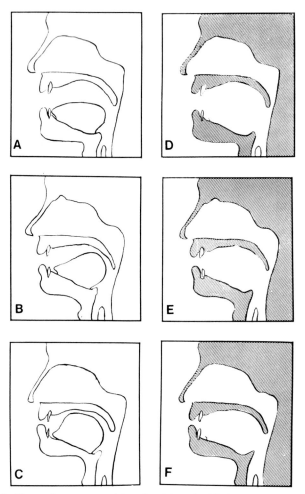

Figure 8. A, Normal tongue position for [a] as in "father." B, Normal tongue position for [u] as in "food." C, Normal tongue position for [i] as in "seen." D, Schema for [a] with tongue excised. E, Schema for [u] with tongue excised. F, Schema for [i] with tongue excised.

The principles to be observed in planning compensations are listed in Table VIII.

The speech wave depends on whether and where the oral cavity is obstructed. The absence of the tongue necessitates a substitute obstructor. This makes it difficult for the glossectomee speaker to produce the fluctuating alterations in the oral cavity size and

TABLE VIII

PRINCIPLES OF CAVITY RESONANCE

Frequency	Volume	Opening	Neck	Lining
higher	smaller	smaller	shorter	more elastic
lower	larger	larger	longer	less elastic

shape usually associated with resonances necessary to specific phonemes. The surgery may also alter the glossectomee's ability to make adequate couplings at optimal speeds.

The clinician judgments proved to be highly correlated with project intelligibility scores and sonagram measures in the project (see Tables IX, X). Other recent studies supported such reliability of clinical opinion. Dillenschneider and his associates (1969) reported that the phoniatrist's ear is still of primary importance, although they presented their method of using the sonagraph to provide an objective picture of dysphonia. Thomas (1969) was even more definite and specific:

> The accuracy and consistency of formant determination using a simple listen and compare method compare favorably with results obtained from more complex analysis procedures.

> Continuous tape loops of vowels were played to listeners who were asked to specify the perceived pitch by comparison with that of a pure-tone oscillator. The perceived pitch of each of the vowels corresponded very closely to F_2 as measured from spectrograms.

TABLE IX

INTELLIGIBILITY SUMMARY
EXPERIMENTAL GROUP

Preproject and Postproject Scores and Mean Measures

Clinician Ranking	Intelligibility Test Scores Norm 100%			Mean K Hz Hi of 7 Glossal Monosyllables Norm 8 K Hz		Mean Duration/Sec of 7 Glossal Monosyllables Norm .52 sec	
	Pre %	Post %	Gain	Pre K Hz	Post K Hz	Pre sec.	Post sec.
1	57	72	15	3.42	6.14	.72	.56
2	55	71	16	2.71	5.00	.59	.54
3	50	66	16	2.92	4.64	.73	.57
4	43	53	10	2.42	4.35	.80	.68
5	34	44	10	2.00	3.28	.76	.68
6	25	35	10	2.50	3.14	.93	.78
7	24	30	6	1.42	2.35	.84	.71
8	20	20	0	0.50	1.42	.27	.27
9	15	15	0	0.50	0.50	.20	.25
10	10	10	0	0.50	0.50	.25	.25

TABLE X

INTELLIGIBILITY SUMMARY
CONTROL GROUP

Preproject and Postproject Scores and Mean Measures

Clinician Ranking	Intelligibility Test Scores Norm 100%			Mean K Hz Hi of 7 Glossal Monosyllables Norm 8 K Hz		Mean Duration/Sec of 7 Glossal Monosyllables Norm .52 sec.	
	Pre %	Post %	Gain	Pre K Hz	Post K Hz	Pre sec	Post sec
1	56	58	2%	3.5	3.5	.72	.72
2	54	56	2%	3.0	3.0	.76	.74
3	51	53	2%	3.0	3.0	.73	.71
4	41	42	1%	2.5	2.5	.80	.80
5	35	36	1%	2.0	2.0	.80	.80
6	27	28	1%	2.5	2.5	.84	.84
7	21	21	None	1.0	1.0	.90	.90
8	20	20	None	.5	.5	.26	.26
9	14	14	None	.5	.5	.25	.25
10	10	10	None	.5	.5	.25	.25

Skelly, Donaldson, Scheer and Guzzardo (1971b) also supported reliability of clinical judgment.

CHANGES IN INTELLIGIBILITY

Comparison of the pretherapy and posttherapy intelligibility scores and the spectrographic shifts in duration and high-frequency measures supported the project hypotheses that there are phonatory aspects of glossectomee intelligibility and that vocal parameter manipulation can increase intelligibility scores (see Tables IX, X).

Such score increase appeared to occur only when there was favorable change in both the measured parameters. When high frequency measure was lower than 3 KHz, the intelligibility score was lower than 50 per cent. The greatest percentage improvement occurred when the high frequency was extended to or above 4 KHz.

Intelligibility was reduced when duration measures were less than the norm or more than twice the norm. One and a half times the norm appeared to be the optimal duration ratio for glossectomees. In therapeutic trials, when duration was reduced below this ratio, regression in score occurred even when the measure still exceeded the norm. The tables indicated some relationship between lower scores and duration decreases beyond the optimal ratio. In the experimental group, the three highest gained 15 per cent, the next three 10 per cent, the 7th 6 per cent, the others none. The three highest of the controls gained 2 per cent, the next three 1 per cent, the others none.

CONCLUSIONS

These higher intelligibility test scores and improvement in life situation communication for the total glossectomee were probably not solely the result of more skillful application by the patient of his articulatory compensations. The intelligibility improvement appeared to have phonatory components, amenable to vocal parameter manipulation.

It was impossible to manipulate one selected parameter of voice, holding all others constant. It was equally futile to ignore phonemic impact. Nevertheless, while clinical manipulation of the vocal parameters with these patients has been thus limited, the results were somewhat encouraging. As in many voice cases, concurrent manipulation of several parameters appeared to accelerate desirable change, with associated (if not consequent) intelligibility improvement. Clinical therapeutic manipulation of the vocal parameters was profitably utilized by encouraging the patient to explore the following:

1. Lengthening of vowel duration.
2. Reduction in vocal intensity (perhaps expressed as tension or muscular effort) .
3. Reduction of rate and intentional use of meaningful pauses.
4. Elevation of the usual abnormally low habitual pitch.
5. Widening of pitch range.
6. Increase in variety of pitch patterning.
7. Perhaps most significantly, improvement in resonance productive of extended harmonic range.

PART THREE

TREATMENT

Chapter VII

PRELIMINARY CONSIDERATIONS IN SPEECH REHABILITATION

AS IN ALL CASES of hospitalized patients, but particularly in post-operative surgical cases, the speech clinician must be aware of the patient's fatigue level. His immediate needs for physical comfort will often dominate the session. The whole course of future progress may depend on the clinician's awareness of the patient's fluctuating physical state. Long-term rehabilitation goals are best served by sensitivity to his immediate discomforts.

The rapport established between patient and clinician in this fashion will enable the latter to provide the support and encouragement so necessary to maintenance of motivation through the long weeks of daily drill required for success. The careful building of the patient's confidence in the clinician's skill and in the patient's own ability to profit from it cannot be overemphasized.

The patient also needs to be cautioned against too early attempts to outrun the therapy goals. Unsuccessful attempts at conversation can be exhausting, discouraging, and frustrating. Family and friends must be included in this orientation if it is to be effective. Expectations must be carefully readjusted. Usually prior to the initiation of the speech clinic schedule, neither patient nor family expect very much in speech. Then with the appearance of the speech clinician, they begin to expect too much. More importantly, they expect it too soon.

It is the latter expectation which may have the greatest adverse effect on progress. Therefore it is very important early in the program to emphasize realistic goals. It is not enough to mention these once in a well-conducted early orientation schedule. Frequent reiteration is needed, especially emphasizing extent of time required for rehabilitation.

The patient and family may have undue expectations regarding the level of restoration to be expected. They almost always underestimate the time necessary to achieve the target goal. Realistic estimates may be so far from this expectation that the patient is very shocked by an abrupt statement on time. It may be helpful to describe the progress made by previous successful patients over certain intervals.

> Mr. M. is at present the most intelligible speaker on our clinic program. His intelligibility score was 12 per cent when he began. Three months later he had progressed to 24 per cent. After six months, he scored 52 per cent. This week, just a year after starting, he has reached 76 per cent so now almost all of his friends understand him, although he still has some problems with strangers.
> Mr. S., who started at zero per cent, progressed in three months to only 12 per cent. At six months, he scored 16 per cent. He and his family almost decided to terminate. In the following three months, he progressed to 20 per cent. When we reevaluated at that time, he wrote:
> "The first time I learned to talk (as a baby) it took me 12 months to get to the first word, so I'm not going to give up yet."
> Three months later, he scored 50 per cent! And he is still improving.

Just as in laryngectomy cases, it is frequently helpful to have a successful glossectomee visit the new patient. This must not be a casual event, however. Rather it must be very carefully planned and even more importantly prepared for in advance, and the visitor cautiously chosen. The temperament and personality of the visitor are important considerations. So far as it is possible to do so, these should match those of the patient. The new patient must be conditioned by adequate information and explanation to accept the facial alterations visually and the speech auditorially.

The attending physician and speech clinician know what great strides the visiting glossectomee has made, so in their evaluation of his present appearance and speech they are comparing the present with admission. The new glossectomee is comparing the visitor with normalcy. Without preparation for a shift in value base, the visit may be traumatic rather than helpful.

A brief sampling by tape recorder of the progress of selected patients at three month intervals over a year's time may be played to the new patient and his family and friends. This has the additional value of preparing the patient's usual listeners for the quality of the improvement, and so adjusting them also to realistic goals. It may also desirably modify some of their communicative conduct with the patient.

It may be very helpful to the patient for the clinician to take the time to inform and condition early visitors. Complete loss of motivation may occur if a friend or relative remarks: "I can't understand a word you said!" On the other hand picking out one clear sequence and asking: "Did you mean top or pop?" may encourage the patient, as well as progressively providing improved communication.

All early counselling should be encouraging and positive. But it is unwise to omit a gradual introduction of negative aspects. Not all motivated, persistent patients succeed in restoring a high intelligibility level. Perhaps the patient's own preoperative speech was far from perfect. This may well be discussed with him. If a preoperative sample recording was obtained, it may be played, commented on, scored on an articulation scale and its rating used as a target for rehabilitation. The patient may have some opinions of the current intelligibility of the various hospital personnel serving him. This will demonstrate that very few, if any, people speak perfectly.

The experienced clinician already has many skills for establishing rapport and motivations. These can be adapted to support the long-term goal in glossectomee rehabilitation of the *restoration of communication,* rather than the perfection of meticulous articulation. After all, even the Bell Telephone Company aims at 50 per cent transmission.

A basic philosophy for rehabilitation in all disability may be summarized in three directives:

1. Emphasize the positive.
2. Accept the negative.
3. Build on the usable.

Characteristically, this philosophy is carried into action in the speech clinic. Efficient, valid testing identifies the positive, negative and usable aspects of the patient's current performance. Too frequently, however, the definition of usable is limited to articulation, a much too narrow concept of human communication.

The transfer of ideas (and emotions) between minds can be accomplished in a wide variety of methods besides the speaking of words. It is important to emphasize this to the glossectomee. He is, of course, already using writing and gestures. The telegraph conveys ideas in combinations of long and short sound tappings. Similarly the heliograph flashes long and short light sequences. The sign language and finger talk of the deaf are in this same "word spelling" category and are non-oral transmission of language.

However, many human communications are achieved despite a *barrier* of language. The American Indians developed a system of hand signals understandable across tribal dialects and useful for communication with the white population, even those who knew no Indian language. The communication systems of smoke signals and drum rhythms used over many continents and by many peoples through many centuries preceded the telegraph and heliograph.

Prior to the introduction of radio transmission, sailors used flags in a series for signaling ideas and still use them in emergency conditions where radio is not practical.

Artists have always conveyed meaning and emotion without words in painting and sculpture. The exquisite dance-mime of the Orient tells a clear story to the foreign observer. The modern interpretative dance of American musicals often clarifies the unintelligibility of the accompanying lyrics. Both the Duncan and the Dunham dancers convey both ideas and emotions. Classic ballet is stylized storytelling. Both music and mathematics use symbol systems without words. The former can convey nuance and the latter exactness utterly beyond language.

Modern life has developed many types of communicative signaling. The red-yellow-green of the traffic light is an example. The new international highway signs are very successful in providing information across language barriers. It is interesting to observe in foreign countries the adaptation of these to hand signals between residents and visitors with no common language.

Some description of all these ingenious inventions of mankind to exchange ideas with his fellow man may encourage the patient in his own compensatory explorations.

Different languages have different sound systems. Although they may share many phonemes, each has some that are unique. The glottal and umlat of German, the characteristic nasals of French and its [oe] as in "boef" and [y] as in "rue" are examples. Spanish has a highly individual [l] as in "calle." Some African languages use teeth clicks while the indrawn breath may be significant for the Oriental tongues.

Just as it is helpful to inform the speechless patient of the numerous alternative methods of human communication, so will the glossectomee gain confidence in his own future speech by information about the variety of language sounds outside the English phoneme repertoire. With proper experimentation, he may be able to produce some of them and to use them as substitutes for the English phonemes he can no longer produce normally.

Different languages have different characteristic tonal, rate and rhythm patterns which help the knowledgeable listener to recognize meaning. Various Amerind and Oriental languages use a certain series of phonemes to convey two or more discrete meanings by distinctive pitch levels. English, too, conveys meaning by tonal inflection patterns. While these are often used intuitively by the native speaker, they are seldom applied intentionally for improvement of intelligibility. Experimentation has indicated that such application is productive, especially for glossectomees.

Many of the immediate aims of therapy may be served by demonstrating the communicative use of tonal patterns with sounds the glossectomee is able to produce, such as a repeated or prolonged [m]. With a rising inflection and continuous phonation pattern, this can mean "What did you say?" or "What do you want?" With a low pitch in a slightly wavering phonation pattern, it can mean "That's nice" or "I like that." Successively interrupted phonations accompanied by increases in intensity produce the equivalent of a wolf whistle and gives the patient the pleasure of surprising a pretty nurse. At a medium pitch, continued to an indefinite fade-out in phonation, it can mean "I don't know" or "I'm not sure." A staccato low-pitch tone phonated twice can indicate an emphatic "No." A single similar high pitch phonation can ask, "Will you?"

Experimentation with this type of tonal language can provide some fun for the patient and at the same time add to his communicative repertoire. It also provides practice in pitch shift which can later improve intelligibility on any achieved glossal compensations.

Both the patient and his friends and family can profit from hints on the use of context clues. We distinguish meaning in this fashion in many instances when the phonemic sequence distorts it in ordinary conversation. Added clues can be gestural or visual. Just as in conversation with the deaf, the glossectomee patient can learn to signal when he changes the subject and so provide a clue for his listeners. He may even plan for conversation with a visitor by preparing printed cue cards to indicate the general subjects he wishes to discuss in order.

Familiarity with a speaker leads a listener to expect certain conditions, vocabulary and even ideas. This can either mislead or assist. Both professionals and family may assume without checking and so frustrate the glossectomee. Or they may anticipate and rob him of the satisfaction of success.

Almost every adult has preconceived and firmly held ideas about his own communicative system. Usually this results in fixed and rigid behaviors in it, somewhat difficult to modify in the clinical situation. The deviant speaker, especially where the change in intelligibility has been a rather sudden consequence of the surgery, perceives the resulting difficulty in understanding as being a property of the listener rather than himself. Frequently the patient reiterates (in writing if necessary) that his wife (or child or friend or doctor) just does not listen! Despite his knowledge of the surgery's consequences, he persists in his prior patterns of speech production and his prior attitudes on the listening habits of others.

With many patients, it will be necessary to convince the individual that his production is not intelligible before he will apply himself adequately to the necessary drills. It has proved useful to collect on tape some of the patient's sentence utterances and to intersplice them with sentences of other glossectomees and other types of dysarthries. The tape can be played for the patient to interpret meaning. Clinical judgment in the individual case will determine whether identification of his own segments will be traumatic. Usually it has been very helpful in enabling the patient to recognize and to accept his current level of intelligibility. This is the first step toward self criticism which must necessarily precede adequate monitoring of speech output for progress.

Regardless of the reported level of education, few patients have knowledge or understanding of phonemic systems or physiologic phonetics. The clinician often errs in use of sophisticated professional terms in providing instruction. The patient is sometimes too proud (or indifferent) to indicate his lack of understanding. When simplified language is inappropriate, possibly the idea may be clarified by a homely illustration or analogy, as well as expanded explanation in colloquial terms. It may help the patient's understanding if instructions given to him in the clinical sessions are repeated to the family members in his presence, rather than conveyed to them privately or separately. It may support his ego if the clinician uses phrases such as, "of course Mr. Blank already knows that . . . ." or "Mr. Blank and I have agreed that . . . ." or "In our session yesterday, Mr. Blank discovered that . . . ." This implies the patient's active and contributory participation in the rehabilitation process as a peer. A teacher-pupil relationship or attitude has no proper place in the treatment of the adult patient.

Each language, in its educational system, has developed standard ways of speech sound production. These have usually been based on the imitation principle: Watch mother, Watch teacher, Do as I do, Listen to Father. The formal study of speech has identified some norms of sound production. In propounding these, it appears that the early speech teachers found it simpler to describe the physiologic method than to explain its acoustic product. In the early years of speech pathology as a profession, when it was designated "speech correction," the method was further refined into meticulous directions for articulator placement, particularly emphasizing the position of the tongue.

In attempting rehabilitation of the speech of the glossectomee, the clinician must be willing to abandon this traditional approach. Both clinician and patient must be willing to believe that while the normal method of phoneme production may be the easiest technique, it is not the only one. Nor is its use the most valid estimate of success. The acoustic result of articulation, what the listener hears and identifies, should be the determiner of success. Compensatory or substitute movements are quite acceptable if they produce the intended sound within phonemic limits such that the average listener can gather the contextual meaning. This implies experimentation with the individual patient's residual articulators.

Unfortunately we Americans are not noted for either the vigor or precision of our articulation. This has positive values for the glossectomee in that his listeners will probably not be overcritical of his deviations. It has negative aspects for the glossectomee in that to his prior imprecision is now added the handicap of surgical alteration of the articulators affecting size, shape, relationships and motility.

It may inspire the patient to try and also encourage him to persist if the limits and directions of the task are defined. He probably already is aware from his own school days that speech sounds are divided into vowels and consonants. If he is an elderly patient, he probably thinks of these alphabetically. If he is phonetically oriented at all, it is probably in terms of long and short vowels and silent and sounded consonants. He may or may not know that discrete language sounds are all called phonemes. By judicious inquiry, the clinician can determine if the patient is aware of the prime differences between vowel and consonant. Does he know that the vowel is usually easier to produce, but also usually less precise? Does he realize that it is an open throat, open mouth, *unimpeded* sound? Does he know that primarily the identity of the individual vowel depends on the size and shape of the oral cavity (mouth) and the size and shape of the opening (lips)? Is he aware that changing the size of the lip opening (and/or its shape) can change the vowel?

The clinician can demonstrate the suggested changes. It may be necessary for the clinician to practice extensively to inhibit the tongue from performing its conditioned responses. One of the narrow wooden tongue depressors can hold the clinician's tongue immobile and let the patient see the mouth and lip changes and hear the acoustic product. It is neither necessary nor desirable in these preliminary instructions to do more than minimal experimentation on vowel production by the patient. At this point, the aim is to convince him that production is possible at an acceptable level and to provide him indirectly with some of the basic information on phonetics.

Does he know that consonants are primarily produced by obstructing the breath stream, by setting up a dam in its flow? The engineer for an electric plant does not really need to care what is used to make a river dam, as long as it efficiently holds back the bulk of the water and directs the overflow to the spillway. Similarly the speaker needs to focus on the damming of the air and the directing of the overflow. The clinician can demonstrate one of the most visible of the consonants usually produced by a tongue-dam: [d] in "do" and "day," then produce this same phoneme in the demonstration word by substituting an inferior labial dam, with the lower lip replacing the tongue tip as the breath-stream obstructor. Previous practice, recording both productions and comparing them, will create confidence in the clinician. Tape-recorded samples of the labial version may be played for the patient to decide their intelligibility. Samples from the speech of other glossectomees may demonstrate the effectiveness of this compensatory approach.

The patient may or may not know that the English language is commonly reported as including forty phonemes. In either case, he probably will not know the hopeful and comforting fact that only eight of these are true "glossal" or tongue sounds. Four of the eight have surd cognates, or sounds articulated in the same pattern but without phonation. Of course the clinician knows that this is ignoring the problem of blends which present so many difficulties for children in the developmental clinic. However, one of the interesting, encouraging and stimulating findings in the early glossectomee studies was the discovery that adult glossectomees do not appear to have any blend problem, as such. Apparently if they master the glossals, they can blend them.

At this stage of the preliminary instruction, the intelligent patient realizes that the mere absence of the tongue mass from his mouth changes the size and may modify the shape of the oral cavity. If he has had a hemimandibulectomy also, he may have some interference with labial movement and control. He knows this will affect the size and shape of the oral cavity opening. The clinician should verbalize these problems.

A demonstration at this time of the effect of articulatory vigor and mandibular excursion can be profitable. With tight jaw and minimal excursion, through flaccid, barely moving lips, at low pitch, in guttural tones, at a rapid rate, the clinician can inform the patient that "At episcopal celebration's the chrysanthemums are usually red, yellow and white." If the clinician's articulators are sufficiently inert, the patient will not be able to understand the message. When it is then repeated with energetic labial and mandibular action, the value of articulatory vigor and jaw movement can be emphasized for future therapeutic drills. The patient can also be prepared for the necessary lip and jaw exercises. He might also at this time be challenged to achieve discrete and reliable control of buccinator movement, drawing the cheeks toward the teeth or gingiva. It has often helped to tell him that most people cannot do this. If he can accomplish such control, it will later help him to form two of the very difficult glossal phonemes [r] and [l].

All of the suggestions presented so far are applicable prior to any formal testing of the patient for therapy planning. In the initial relationship postoperatively, it is advisable to visit the patient briefly. Three 10-minute visits in a day appear to be more effective than a single 30-minute one. Frequency of contact may be much more important at this time than length of session. If only one of the preliminary informational topics is covered in a visit, the patient has time to think it over before the clinician returns. If he has questions, he has opportunity to prepare them in writing. Whether or not he presents queries, the prior topic should be reviewed before the new one is presented.

A few days of such conditioning of the patient and of his family and friends can be very profitable in enhancing rapport and in motivation, providing a favorable climate for progress, determining the patient's individual immediate needs and adjusting him and his associates to realistic goals for rehabilitation. During these informal sessions, the clinician has opportunity to glean a knowledge of the patient's attitudes and reactions that provides a solid base for formal testing.

Chapter VIII

THERAPY: TESTING

Formalized test procedures have three major purposes:

1. To provide detailed, organized data on the individual patient in areas pertinent to diagnosis, prognosis and treatment.
2. To facilitate comparison with similar cases and with normative data.
3. To measure progress in treatment.

None of these intentions is well served unless the test data are scrutinized against a background of knowledge of the

1. Particular patient's individual differences from all other patients in terms of age, medical history, etiological factors, education, intelligence, personality, motivation, employment, family, finances, etc.
2. Specifics of his disability (such as surgical alteration, muscle and neural impairment or residual deficits).

Prior to scheduling of formal testing but concurrent with the preliminary visits described in the previous chapter, the clinician needs to acquire and correlate a wide variety of information about the patient. The family (or friends) may be able to provide a great deal. The advice and assistance of other professional personnel may also be needed.

The economic consequences of cancer and surgery may weigh heavily on the patient's spirits and the family's attitudes. The psychological impact of disability and deformity must be estimated. The patient's emotions, prior life, employment, needs and aspirations are all relevant. The extent of his prior social life may be a critical factor in his successful adaptation. His education and intelligence are highly related to his problem-solving behaviors and to his attitudes in therapy.

The Leiter Scale of non-verbal measurement of learning and problem-solving abilities has proved very helpful in assessing speechless patients in speech clinic evaluation. Its results are most useful if the speech clinician administers it or at least observes its administration. The psychologist may find the scoring of major importance, but the speech clinician can also use the patient's behavior in the tasks to great advantage. Many deductions for effective therapy planning may develop from observation of the method and order of attack the patient uses on the test tasks. The test also reveals specifics on visual deficits and imperceptions and provides data on motor coordination, self-correction and speed of processing.

The clinician should scan the medical chart and abstract pertinent data. The surgery in each case may dictate specific adjustment of both goals and methods of both testing and treatment. The exact anatomical, physiological and innervation alterations must be recorded and analyzed for their impact on form and shape, muscle movement and control for this particular patient.

Only against the coherent total current picture of the individual patient as a whole person can formal speech testing serve its purported intent. Extensive testing of any sick person must justify itself by serving his personal and individual needs.

Prior to the formal test session (or sessions) it is wise to use the tape recorder with the patient in informal interviews, particularly if he is elderly. There is little doubt of the value of taping the test sessions. This provides a permanent record of the patient's status and behavior on admission. It also supports progress reports through comparison with periodic tape samples and termination recordings at discharge. It permits consultation with other professionals in scoring and evaluation. It allows the clinician to examine repeatedly what is but a monetary acoustic event in memory otherwise. Familiarizing the patient with the routine prior to formal examination helps to prevent any bias in his responses due to the presence of the instrument.

Experience indicates the advisability of dictating the patient's name, hospital identification, the date of the testing and the examiner's name directly onto the tape. External labeling is frequently lost. If possible, maintenance of standard testing conditions will provide greater reliability and validity in the testing. The ambient noise level, the specifications of tape recorder and the microphone, the recording level and the distance from the patient's lips to microphone should be standardized. These standards may well be printed or typed on the test form. Any departures from the usual standards and procedures should be noted on the report of results. When data are recorded, the chart should indicate whether they are derived from clinician judgments or instrumental measurements, such as pitch meter, sound pressure meter, spectrograph, audiometer, speech audiometer, etc.

It usually facilitates the patient's normal response level if testing begins with conversation. So the first test task consists of questions and answers. Both are recorded. This provides a basis for speech energy comparisons of the clinician's voice and the patient's replies.

Normally a person's conversational speech changes in a number of parameters when he reads aloud. A brief sample from "Arthur the Rat" has been incorporated in the glossectomee test battery rather than any of the widely accepted, more adult selections in the literature, in order to avoid as far as possible distortions due primarily to reading competence.

If the patient cannot read for any reason and must repeat after the clinician, it is helpful to rehearse before recording so that the patient's recorded responses do not reflect any difficulty in following the clinician. (There is no intent to test auditory memory at this stage in the test. The clinician should depress the hold lever during his presentation so that his voice is not included in the sample.

It is helpful for the vision of sick people if the printed stimuli are typed in the large print of a primer typewriter or hand-blocked in large letters on cards.

Since vowels are anatomically and physiologically easier to produce than consonants, they may well measure for the tester the patient's best phoneme production. Since extended duration has been demonstrated to improve intelligibility, the so-called long vowels are designated as the test items. The elderly patient also recognizes this type of classification. There is little to be gained at this point in the patient's program in exploring the vowel triangle. It is enough for diagnosis and prognosis to explore his ability to produce distinguishable or identifiable long vowels [e], [i], [aɪ], [o] and [u]. By a score of distinguishable is meant that the sounds are obviously different from one another, although not sufficiently within phonemic limits to be discretely identified.

The patient should then be requested to repeat his best vowel, holding it as long as one breath permits. This should be timed and the number of seconds entered as the resonant duration. He should then have the sound [f] demonstrated (but not named) and asked to hold it as long as possible. It should be measured only after he has practiced. Similarly, [v] should be demonstrated, practiced and timed. The seconds are entered respectively for sonant and surd duration. The timing of any quavers should be noted, as quavered production is not normal. The norm for each (resonant, sonant, surd) is approximately 18 seconds. Many healthy young people and almost all athletes, trained speakers, actors and singers score much higher. Scores below 14 for adults are alerting signals for pulmonary and/or laryngeal difficulties. If a score falls below 18, three trials should be made and recorded.

If the three differ, an irregular pattern may indicate possible problems in innervation and/or muscle control and coordination. If the scores present a descending pattern, the patient may be fatiguing. In either of these cases, it may be advisable to terminate the test and schedule its completion the next day, repeating this segment of the test for reliability of obtained scores.

A rising pattern indicates a favorable prognosis both for improved phonatory control and also for speech intelligibility.

The next test task requests the patient to produce any sound, preferably the open vowel [ɑ], at his highest pitch, then at his lowest pitch. Next he is asked to glide from lowest to highest without halting phonation, then the same from highest to lowest. Finally, he is directed to produce the lowest, halt phonation, and then at once produce the highest, and to replicate the last in the reverse direction, from highest to lowest. Analysis of his successes and failures, as well as duration, pause intervals, direction and ease of shift, provide insights on extent and speed of laryngeal control. The easiest shifts become the usable components in therapeutic modifications.

In the next test item, the patient is asked to combine the non-glossal consonants with the vowels in CV and VC patterns so we may assess this limited production and contrast it with his similar CV and VC patterns with attempts at the glossal consonants.

The next task is the speaking of the non-glossal word list, then the non-glossal sentences. The next item is the glossal word list, then the glossal sentences. Summation is made of any success differences between the non-glossal items and the glossal tasks.

The next segment of the speech testing utilizes four words from the non-glossal list. The patient records all four—"foam," "wipe," "heap," "pave." He is then asked to repeat each word under the following circumstances:

1. With greater muscular vigor (labial).
2. With wider jaw excursion (mandibular).
3. At faster speed (rate).
4. At slower speed (rate).
5. With jaw moving forward (thrust).
6. At a high pitch (frequency).
7. With vowel prolongation (duration).
8. With increased loudness (intensity).

If spectrography is available, spectrograms of these 32 utterances may be printed and analyzed for the effect of the directives. In any case, the clinician is expected to evaluate any changes. Desirable shifts may be incorporated for use in treatment.

Either at this time or as soon as possible, an audiological test is scheduled. The usual treatment should follow for any hearing deficits that are identified. Speech approaches will need to be adapted to suit any hearing loss. The patient's discrimination score is particularly relevant to the speech rehabilitation. If he has discrimination problems, they will seriously interfere with his progress in developing useful compensations. Auditory judgment and monitoring of the adequacy of the acoustic result of the compensations is basic to stabilization of the compensatory synergy.

The discrimination testing is most conveniently accomplished with tape recorder stimulus, since this can be halted manually.

Since the patient cannot speak, he must, of course, be given time to write what he hears. This procedure will consume more time and effort than checking one of a pair of printed words or identifying one of a group of pictures. It is worth the additional time and effort if it indicates any problem. It is particularly valuable if it identifies any subtle confusions in discrimination, since these are seldom apparent in the results of the binary choice check type of test. The patient's auditory memory span is relevant and should be checked.

All the materials presented thus far have implied the clinician's authority and competence to make the test judgments. That this is a valid assumption is supported by many studies. Yet several that support it also show that the clinician ranking agrees with other ranking, but clinicians tend to award consistently (but proportionately) higher scores than other methods produce.

The speech clinic is interested in test scores only as valid diagnostic, prognostic or progress measures. Learning theory proposes that involvement in process accelerates learning. It may be wise to involve the patient early in self-evaluation, since one clinical goal should be adequate development of self-judgment and self-correction. Listening to his own test or therapy tapes critically is a worthwhile learning activity. At least a few sessions with adequate controls should be set up to test his reliability before he is permitted to listen, exercising subjective judgment only. The clinician may find it profitable to take time to make some spliced tapes for reliability listening, intersplicing the patient's efforts among those of others. Incidentally, the recording and judging of such intersplices are valuable activities for students in professional training in the clinic.

The same spliced tapes may be used for further and different scoring contributing to validation of both clinician and patient judgment. Many hospital visitors with waiting time on their hands will willingly participate briefly in tape listening and judging. This is also a method of interesting and (even educating) various hospital personnel in the speech clinic. It is not difficult to interest students at nearby college and university programs in such judgmental listening. Many professionals are eager to extend their knowledge of glossectomee speech by participating.

If clinician-patient-visitor triple scoring of tests occurs, correlations should be determined and included in the report. Admission and discharge testing are understandably the two most important. Monthly and quarterly measures of progress assist in clinical planning. Sometimes weekly or even daily scoring of specific activities may be highly motivating to the patient.

The admissions test for glossectomee patients currently in use at the St. Louis Veterans Administration Hospital Audiology and Speech Pathology Service is included in the Appendix. It may be reproduced for use by any operating clinic with a professional staff. It has, of course, not been standardized and is still in process of development, adjustment and improvement. Nevertheless in its present form it provides a record of the patient's speech behavior in certain parameters under certain circumstances. It is devised to yield useful information for design of treatment.

Section A yields a brief sample of the patient's current intelligibility level in a minimally structured situation. It provides cues for the listener in the questions. It assesses the patient's ability to convey life situation information. It is a quick assessment of his communicability rather than intelligibility.

Section B yields material for the usual articulation scoring of continuous speech in a contextual frame, on a prose segment widely accepted as test material. It explores (in the complete form) all the English phonemes. It permits identification of any substitution the patient is making for the glossal consonants. It provides opportunity for comparison of the patient's speech on free response to questions (Item A) and his speech when reading assigned material (Item B), both in phonetic and phonatory parameters.

Section C includes a sentence containing all the glossal consonants. It explores all the non-glossal consonants and includes most of the vowels. It provides a record of initial aspirate influence. This segment alone may be used for many purposes, such as spectrographic sampling, monthly sample recording and scoring. It may also be substituted for the longer examination at the discretion of the clinician with certain patients, especially those who fatigue quickly. Spectrographic analysis and/or repeated listening to this tape-recorded brief form can yield much usable information.

Section D explores the patient's vocal pitch range and control. It provides information which can be used in parameter manipulation in therapy. It guides the clinician's expectation concerning the patient's fine muscular synergies.

It supplies additional information on glottal control efficiency. It indicates possible problem areas in breath pressure control and phonation contrasts between open and obstructed phonation. This information is important in clinic planning, as it guides choice of word lists, so that the most difficult materials are not presented to the patient too early in his program.

Section E serves the same purpose with special application to the very early sessions. The patient's "best" or "easiest" vowel is always the desirable choice for early drills. It is advisable to have the patient himself participate in rating many of the test items in these terms.

Section F provides sampling of the eight glossal consonants under consideration in early therapy planning. They are presented in isolated words in the initial position (except [ŋ] of course). This position appeared easiest for the patient's first attempts. The vowel [o] has been used for the testing because it appeared to be the easiest for the majority of the glossectomees to produce differentially. The words are listed in the test in the order of difficulty (from easiest to most difficult) evolved in the St. Louis Veterans Administration Clinic. The examiner may wish to note whether or not the patient under test has any different order of difficulty. The [ŋ] provides opportunity to assess effect of varying preceding vowels on its final position.

Sections G and H provide word sampling of the patient's intelligibility in materials lacking glossal consonants. If these sections yield a high intelligibility score, as contrasted with a much lower score on standard testing, the prognosis for intelligibility improvement is usually very favorable.

The word list lends itself to random rearrangement for successive quick brief testing. Its segments are short enough for acoustic spectrography sampling and comparison.

Section I explores the effects of specific physiologic and phonatory manipulations on each of four words for clinical planning deductions. Successive spectrography of these same words at periodic intervals provides objective support of any observed phonatory shifts.

Section J provides a sampling across all the English phonemes and so may be used for comparisons with Section H. The Everyday Sentences are available in eight forms and so provide material for successive monthly testing and comparison of scores.

Section K provides for brief assessment by the clinician of the effects of vocal parameter manipulations which may be used profitably for change.

The final judgments on items and the subsequent summary of the test results should evolve from several sessions of tape listening. Many very profitable insights into problems and applicable remedial techniques accrue from "second hearing."

Chapter IX

THERAPY: PROCEDURES

GOAL SETTING

THE ESTABLISHMENT of target goals is the first item in efficient clinical planning. Overly optimistic expectations of achievement are usually productive only of disappointment and frustration. It is easy and also encouraging and gratifying to extend goals upward on the basis of achievement. The identification of subgoals and especially the arrangement of their hierarchical progression are probably the most important and creative of the clinician's functions. No textbook prescription suffices. Here the qualified professional makes a unique contribution to the treatment of each individual patient.

Provision should be made in the planning for periodic reassessment of goals in terms of the passage of time and the progress of the patient. Decisions concerning the total ongoing rehabilitation plan and any modifications of the original version must be made on the basis of these reevaluations in combination with the individual's needs in his life situation.

This is accomplished most efficiently and effectively if the criteria for the needs, goals, progress and discharge are determined as early as possible after the admission testing and a reasonable period of exploratory therapy. Each professional clinician can choose on this basis for each individual patient among the suggestions that follow.

A BASIC CLINICAL PATTERN

Just as in the human being's early childhood acquisition of language, the glossectomee's development of compensatory speech must be preceded by purposeful listening and effective auditory discrimination. Adults listen to meanings rather than to sounds.

104

The impaired adult speaker must first relearn sound listening. It is easier to focus in the beginning on the sound production of others and then to adapt the skill to self-listening. The latter is best accomplished with the aid of a tape recorder. Some of the other speech reproducers such as the Language Master, Echorder, tape loop and Canon Repeat Corder may focus attention more effectively and accomplish learning more swiftly by limiting the quantity of the stimulus.

Comparison of sound productions follows as a logical second step. The patient should have definite assignments in comparing the speech of those around him in the hospital environment such as medical staff, other hospital employees, other patients, visitors, etc. When his judgment has been validated on others, the patient may compare his own attempts with patterns provided by the clinician. The patient probably needs direction in separating the comparing skill from the matching step which follows. During the comparing step, the task is solely one of auditory judgment. At this stage, the decision should be binary, indicating only that the output is or is not comparable to the stimulus. The patient should be listening at this point to other normal speakers in life situations. The patient's attempts to match his own output to the clinicians pattern should be concentrated entirely on evaluation rather than on perfection of the output.

Eventually the exercises in effective listening, discriminative comparison and accurate matching summate in the desirable self-monitoring which is an essential prerequisite to successful compensatory production. Not until these listening skills have been adequately developed should the clinician permit attempts at compensation with focus on the production.

This second clinical stage should begin, not with emphasis on articulation within phonemic limits, but rather on an exploratory, free-wheeling experimentation. If possible, this should be an amusing and interesting experience for the patient, encompassing all the sounds, speech or otherwise, that the human face, throat and adjacent cavities are capable of making. Glossectomees who have had no oral communication for some time are both delighted and encouraged by the successful production of a raspberry. This early physiological experimentation should include unorthodox movements and combinations not ordinarily used in normal speech synergies. This exercise yields useful information concerning possible compensatory combinations. Even more importantly, it convinces the patient that numerous sounds can be produced in unusual ways. Both are necessary bases for progress.

Among the sounds produced in this exploratory step many can be associated with specific phonemes. After such identification, drills may be undertaken to establish them within acceptable phonemic limits. Thus, kinetic reinforcement will also accrue. The patient's attention should be focused on awareness of muscle movement, awareness of size and shape changes, awareness of contriction agent and locus.

Adequate drill is a necessary concomitant of progress. It is natural and human for the patient who has had some small success to want to push forward to the next step without sufficient drill to stabilize each level of achievement. The clinical consequence is very often a regression in the hard-won intelligibility level with ensuing discouragement and frustration.

Each stage of the intelligibility progress effected by compensatory articulation may be enhanced by systematic vocal parameter manipulation. Clinical planning here may profitably list each parameter variation as a separate subgoal task. Attention may thus be directed to the specific shift which produces any desirable change. Those which are ineffective may be discarded early from the individual program.

As the unprofitable approaches are weeded out and the profitable isolated for use, goal emphasis may shift to the establishment of control, auditory and kinetic. Both are necessary to effect the reliable replication of successes that lead to stabilization of phonemic production. Here again, the amount of drill bears a high relationship to the progress. Each patient has his own individual pattern of fatigue, tolerance and motivation. Numerous daily brief sessions on a regularly scheduled basis are usually more productive than a single lengthy session. With many patients, ten-minute drills every hour can be encouraged by placing the assignments on a "job" basis. This is his daily work. Measures of productivity should be determined jointly by patient and clinician. They may often be related to the patient's former occupation in a highly motivating manner. At the same time, they may yield reinforcement as a measure of accomplishment.

Additional reinforcement may be provided by some previously agreed upon method of having the clinician give approval of the addition of new words to the vocabulary for use in the patient's daily life situations. This application of the clinical goals of the daily sessions may provide a quite adequate method of integrating the day by day improvements into the total communicative behavior of the patient.

Outline of Techniques

I. Initial modification of habitual behaviors.
  A. Telegraphic writing.
  B. Oral rephrasing.
II. Listening.
  A. Identification of sounds.
  B. Discrimination among similar sounds.
  C. Recognition of sound variants within phonemic limits.
  D. Monitoring speech of other glossectomees.
  E. Self-evaluation of intelligibility.
III. Speaking
  A. Manipulation modes.
    1. Behavior manipulation—consistency in substitution.
    2. Physiologic manipulation—muscle exercises for control and excursion.
    3. Phonatory manipulation.
  B. Phonemic modes—normal and compensatory.
    1. Vowels.
      a. Buccal movement.
      b. Mandibular thrust.
      c. Mandibular elevation.
      d. Labial aperture alterations.
      e. Tape recording monitoring.
      f. Exploration of shift combinations.
      g. Visual reinforcement of shift.
      h. Contrasted vowel shifts.
      i. Vowel words.
      j. Attitude change.

   2. Consonants.
     a. Nonglossal.
       1) Ballistic drill on VC combinations.
       2) Analysis of daily speech needs.
       3) Flip cards.
       4) Gestural cues.
       5) Amerind sign.
       6) Phonatory manipulation.
     b. Glossal sounds—normal and compensatory.
       2) [d] [t].
       2) [z] [s].
       3) [n].
       4) [g] [k].
       5) [l].
       6) [r].
       7) [ŋ].
       8) [ð] [θ].
       9) Phonatory manipulation.
       10) Glossal summary.
     c. Consonant review

Specific Technique

I. *Modification of habitual behavior.*

Most adults appear to have two communicative habits which are rather firmly fixed as part of the mature communicative pattern. The first is the determination to be complete in all written communication. The second is the tendency toward simple reiteration when the listener does not understand. The first two specific directives are intended to modify these habits to produce speedier and less frustrating immediate improvement.

  A. *Telegraphic writing.*

This skill may be described and illustrated. The patient may be requested to do all his communicative writing in a pocket notebook instead of a pad, so materials from daily life situations become the basis of drill for change. Each day's written output should then be rewritten as an exercise. The patient is instructed to say the same thing in the irreducible minimum number of words. The older patient may need the definite statement that sentences are not required here. They are not necessary in his daily contacts. He should also learn to stop writing as soon as the listener indicates he has received (or guessed) the message. Numerous patients continue to insist on completing the full written text on an idea even after the listener has demonstrated his reception by replying. It is almost as if the patient, deprived of his normal oral approach, is determined to demonstrate a superior ability in the written mode. The goal in each communication event is transmission of the idea in the fewest possible words, omitting all the unnecessary words such as "the," "and," "but," etc. Progress scores can be made in terms of the difference between the number of words the patient can eliminate and the number the clinician can eliminate. When these numbers coincide consistently, the patient has probably mastered telegraphic writing.

Mastery of telegraphic writing accelerates daily communication almost immediately. It also tends to reduce the patient's complete dependence on the written word. It encourages him to use the telegraphic form merely as a supplement to the oral.

It has an additional advantage should the patient be unable to develop a useful level of compensatory intelligibility. Telegraphic writing prepares the way for the phrasing basic to the manual Indian Sign some speechless patients have found useful.
B. *Oral rephrasing.*

During his early postoperative attempts at speaking, the patient habitually persists in mere repetition when he is not understood. This evokes pity rather than comprehension in the listener. It usually results in frustration in the glossectomee, even developing into anger at the listener.

A unit demonstrating the profits gained by *rephrasing* rather than repeating can be very helpful. It not only improves the immediate situation but has lasting results in directing the patient's attention to the need for awareness of the listener's problems in comprehending. The glossectomee can be educated to attend to both overt and subtle feedback from the listener. Successful communication is significantly related to this awareness of the listener's reactions in confirming reception of the message the speaker is sending. In the drills, the clinician can choose specific phrases for pretended non-comprehension. The patient then responds by rephrasing. The clinician can gradually require two, then three, rephrasings before responding and so perfect the patient's skills in rephrasing habitually.

The patient should keep a cumulative list of the occasions requiring repetitions and also of the successful rephrasings. This is helpful in vocabulary modification and extension. It is also useful for weekly analysis of any lack of progress, by specifically identifying exact problem phonemes or combinations. Some combinations are more difficult to understand as well as to speak. The glossectomee succeeds with "home," has some difficulty with "house" and is usually not understood when he uses "residence."

II. *Listening.*

A. *Identification of sounds.*

An initial unit of word pairs differing in only one phoneme should be presented to the patient for identification of the differing phonemes. Usually the initial position is easiest, the final next, and the middle most difficult. When the patient understands the task and has achieved success with the clinician's help, he can be assigned automated programmed drill with tape recorder or Language Master with prepared response sheets which he checks for the clinician to monitor his output.

B. *Discrimination among similar sounds.*

Paired lists may be presented here first by live voice and then on tape to improve the patient's discrimination of easily confused sounds. On the drills he might be assigned to write suitable short sentences as a response to cassette auditory stimulation.

C. *Recognition of sound variants (within phonemic limits).*

Short tapes of connected speech recorded by persons with various speech handicaps form a useful tool in the speech clinic. The patient may be assigned short listening periods requiring him to write what he hears. The samples may increase in listener difficulty or they may be paired as contrast of extremes. Both arrangements are useful. This type of listener tape should not be concentrated solely on the speech of glossectomee patients. Various dysarthrias and dyslalias should be represented. Samples of colloquial, regional and dialectical variants which sometime interfere with communication may also be profitably utilized as well as monitoring the errors of other glossectomees.

Much of the material in speech-reading manuals provides selections for recording for discriminatory listening drills. Occasional samples by speakers with clear enunciation should be included. The individual patient's specific discrimination problems can be selectively emphasized. The clinician may prepare tapes with clear enunciation except for specific, purposefully chosen variants.

D. *Monitoring speech of other glossectomees.*

In untreated glossectomee speech, random substitutions tend to recur. Short passages may be clipped from recordings of several prior patients. The new patient listens and writes what he hears. His subgoals may include assignments for identifications of specific substitutions or consistent and inconsistent substitutions as well as ratings of various substitutions on an intelligibility scale.

E. *Self-evaluation of intelligibility.*

The patient's attempts to speak are tape recorded cumulatively during the period spent on the approaches outlined so far. Now he listens to them critically. The recordings are enough in the past that he will not clearly and accurately remember the content. He listens for his own general intelligibility, identifies his substitutions and evaluates their consistency.

III. *Speaking.*

A. *Manipulation.*

1. *Behavior manipulation—consistency in substitution.*

Most glossectomees substitute some of the nonglossal for the glossal sounds in their daily communication. Many times, however, these are not produced with desirable differentiation. Neither are they used with consistency. It may be advantageous to the patient's daily communication to spend some time at this point developing differentiation and consistency. The most frequently used substitutions are as follows:

[v–f] are substituted for [s–z]
[d–t]
[θ–ð]

[ɟ] is substituted for [d–t]

$$[g\text{--}k]$$
[w] and/or [a] for [r] and [ɝ]
[j] or [w] for [l]
[n] or [ȵ] or [nȵ] for [ŋ]

It is apparent at once from the above list that the patient should be encouraged to be consistent to avoid compounding the confusion already existing. It has proved most profitable to date to establish consistency as:

[v–f] substituting only for [ð–θ]
[ȵ]   ″   ″   ″   [g–k]
[w]   ″   ″   ″   [r]
[ɜ]   ″   ″   ″   [ɝ]
[j]   ″   ″   ″   [l]
[nȵ]   ″   ″   ″   [ŋ]
air puff   ″   ″   ″   [z–s]

In a great many cases, many months may elapse before the patient can develop adequate compensations. Time and effort spent at this point in his therapy on *consistent* substitutions can provide him the dignity of useful, even though distorted, communication.

In addition to the auditory training and behavioral modifications already suggested, procedures and techniques may be grouped in two broad categories: (a) physiologic manipulation for compensatory articulation and (b) phonatory manipulation of the vocal parameters. Both of these are applied to three broad phonetic groupings: vowels, non-glossal consonants and glossal sounds. The phonatory manipulations have proved most profitable when applied after development of adequate physiologic adaptation so discussion of its applications follows the segments on glossal consonants.

2. *Physiologic manipulation—muscle exercises for control and excursion.*

The parameters involved include

Labial			
Mandibular		cavity	size
Buccal	modifications		shape
Pharyngeal	in relation to	orifice	couplings
Sphincteric			size
			shape
		movement	vigor
			excursion
			direction

In each individual case, the clinician will plan a suitable series of indicated muscular exercises to improve control of the modifications and relationships indicated. A triptych mirror will enable the patient to observe the lateral as well as frontal effect of his attempts at such modification. Video taping, if available, serves the added advantage of more objective observation by the patient. He can concentrate on observation alone rather than dividing his attention with the pressures and anxieties of production. It enables the patient to view the past event rather than the one in progress. More specific applications of physiologic manipulation follow in relation to the phonetic categories.

3. Phonatory manipulation.

(Listed following the phonemic modes)

B. *Phonemic modes—normal and compensatory.*

1. *Vowels.*

Phoneticians are agreed that it is difficult to describe the positions and movements necessary for the production of the vowels. The very essence of a vowel is a certain openness. This essential characteristic inevitably produces imprecision.

Six moving segments of the anatomy are usually considered available for normal alteration of the size and shape of the oral and pharyngeal cavities. Vowel modification is thus effected by movement of the lips, jaw, tongue, velum, epiglottis and larynx. The tension of the articulatory apparatus is also important in subtle differentiations of the acoustic output. No one of these articulatory agents is indispensable in the production of acceptable vowel sounds.

Rather than any definitive position for successful production of a specific phoneme, a range of relationships should be considered. It may be profitable to review the normal production and contrast it with compensatory modification.

In normal production of the front vowels, the [i] is a high, front, tense, spread vowel. The corners of the mouth are pulled somewhat lateralward. The tongue is arched forward in the mouth. Its highest point is forward of the central apex of the hard palate. It is close but not in actual contact with the hard palate. This results in a division of the oral space into a small anterior cavity and a larger posterior cavity. The mandible is lowered slightly. The lips are open.

This is considered the highest of the front vowel series consisting of [i], [ɪ], [e], [ɛ], [æ] and [a]. Normal differentiation among these vowels rests primarily on locus of the highest arched portion of the tongue. The arch moves posteriorly and inferiorly as the series progresses from [i] to [a]. The lips open more widely in the progression and change from the characteristic [i] spread to a more and more round relationship. The throat is usually tense for [i] and [e] and lax with the other front vowels.

In normal production of the back vowels, the [u] is the highest, back, tense vowel. The lips are rounded and somewhat protruded. The tongue is arched high and posteriorly. A narrow passageway between the pharynx and tongue is thus created through which the sound must pass with consequent modification. The jaw position does not appear to be critical.

The arching of the tongue is lower and lower and shifts slightly posteriorly as one moves from [u] through [u], [o], [ɔ], [ɒ] to [a] while the lips are less and less rounded.

    a. *Buccal movement.*

In clinical approaches with surgical patients (both glossectomees and laryngectomees) , some voluntary movements of the cheeks have been acquired by a number of patients through sucking and blowing routines. The cheek movement appears to contribute to some phonemes compensatorially.

    b. *Mandibular thrust.*

A forward movement of the mandible or remaining segment of the altered mandible appears to be significantly related to vowel differentiation in intelligible glossectomee speech.

    c. *Mandibular elevation.*

Tilting the head back with consequent elevation of the mandible and tensing of the neck appears to contribute to the subtle control of vowel difference for many patients.

    d. *Labial aperture alterations.*

The glossectomee achieving reliable discrete vowels appears to accomplish this primarily by modifying the size and shape of the labial aperture.

e. *Tape recording monitoring.*

Record the patient's attempt to produce the vowels within phonemic limits. The patient judges his own output.

f. *Exploration of shift combinations.*

Compare the sound changes under the following directives:

    1) Adduct the lips until they are almost touching laxly.
        a) Phonation is sustained.
        b) Phonation is interrupted into short, sharp grunts.
    2) Repeat with the lip corners stretched as widely as possible.
    3) Repeat, moving the lips from the almost closed lax position to as wide an abduction vertically as possible.
    4) Repeat with the lips rounded, when the aperture is as follows:
        a) As small as possible.
        b) As large as possible.
        c) Changes from small to large.
        d) Changes from large to small.
    5) Repeat all above and add lip eversion where possible.
    6) Repeat all the above and add mandibular thrust.
    7) Repeat all the above and add head tilt.

g. *Visual reinforcement of shift.*

Patient observation of clinician demonstration, patient mirror observation of his own shifts, video observation of his own and those of others reinforce both the auditory monitoring and the kinetic feedback on vowel successes.

h. *Contrasted vowel shifts.*

Pair widely contrasting vowels:

[a] to [i]
[a] to [o]
[i] to [o]

Note changes resulting from more vigorous lip movement, more vigorous jaw movement, thrusting the jaw forward on phonation, and tilting the head backward on phonation.

i. *Vowel words.*

An early session on vowel production drill may be terminated profitably by demonstrating to the patient that vowel clarity efforts are productive of improved communication for daily use. Words can now be substituted for head shaking. Since the latter is not always easy for the glossectomee postoperatively, progress is evident to him when [iɛ] or [ie] may be used for "yes" and a nasalized [o] for "no."

j. *Attitude change.*

The speech clinician as well as the patient has some preconceived ideas and well-established attitudes requiring some modification with surgical patients. With the total glossectomee, particularly, efforts to replicate the customary approaches of articulation therapy are ineffective. Speech rehabilitation for the total glossectomee cannot be regarded as articulation therapy. In glossectomee rehabilitation, the problem is not one of indicating what is normal and assisting the normal mouth to achieve it. The patient presumably has had at least adequate articulation preoperatively. Neither is the problem actually one of helping him to regain his preoperative articulation which is now anatomically and physiologically impossible. The real goal is acquisition of compensatory or substitute conditions what can produce acceptable acoustic results. The speech clinician, as well as the patient, must accept this goal and the attitude changes needed to achieve it.

2. The Consonants.

Consonant sounds are normally achieved physiologically through the action of variable valves which modify the exhaled breath stream for speech. These valves are functionally created by contact of:

    a. The vocal bands at the glottis.

    b. The soft palate and the pharynx.

c. The tongue and soft palate.
d. The tongue and hard palate.
e. The tongue and superior alveolar ridge.
f. The tongue and superior teeth.
g. The lower lip and superior teeth.
h. The lips in relation to each other.

These valves close, constrict or open the channels through which the expired air passes. Acceptable acoustic patterns of the consonants depend to a considerable extent on the modifications of pressure so effected. A number of phoneticians suggest or imply that the locus of the valving is the most significant factor in consonant production. But in the compensatory approach, it is important only to the extent that an adaptation affects acceptable phonemic limits in the acoustic result. This is supported in the literature by copious references to a number of compensatory valvings noted in the clinical setting in patients with a range of speech problems other than those resulting from glossectomy. Three serve as examples:

a. A frequently observed adaptation for [g] is tongue contact with the posterior pharyngeal wall rather than the velum.
b. When the palatopharyngeal port fails to make adequate closure, a substitute valve may be created by pinching the nares.
c. Dysphonia plica ventricularis is actually a substitute adduction of the ventricular valve for that of the vocal bands.

This is not to imply that the glossectomee should occlude the nares or develop ventriculosis. The pharyngeal approach to the [g], however, may be useful. The important message from these clinical deviations is that recognizable consonantal phonemes may be produced by unorthodox valving when the normal or usual occlusion is unavailable to the patient.

In the list of the eight valve contacts usually considered as producing the consonants of English, only four specifically list the tongue. The others rely primarily upon the lips for

differentiation. For the purpose of glossectomee rehabilitation, consonants therefore are grouped into glossal and non-
glossal consonants.

   a. *Nonglossal consonants.*

   It is neither necessary nor desirable to postpone consideration of the non-glossal consonants until the total
vowel triangle has been mastered. Many normal speakers in
a number of geographic areas do not clearly distinguish the
central vowels. The clinician should judge in the individual
case the optimum moment at which to add the non-glossal
consonants, either postponing or integrating further vowel
drill. The non-glossal consonants combined with the patient's clear vowels will facilitate formation of useful words,
a highly desirable and motivating step at this point.

   1) *Ballistic drill on VC combinations.*

   Non-glossal consonants may be added to the stabile
vowels. Unless there has been severe impairment of the
lips, the following consonants can be produced with
apparent ease and high intelligibility by the glossectomee,
if the previously suggested drills on vigor and excursion
have been carried out: [b], [f], [h], [j], [m], [p], [v], and
[w].

   These are organized in CV, VC, CVC, and VCV combinations to facilitate the patient's first attempts at join-
ing two sounds ballistically. This approach produces some
meaningful monosyllabic words. After a brief initial use,
the nonsense syllable approach should be abandoned
with the adult patient. Only those phoneme combinations which result in meaningful words should be retained for further drill. Adult male patients, particularly, appear to resent the nonsense approach and to label
it childish.

   2) *Analysis of daily speech needs.*

   At this stage of the patient's progress, it is advisable to
eliminate as many as possible of his unintelligible utterances while encouraging him to use those which are
understandable to the listener. An analysis of his daily

speech needs is useful. It provides a realistic subgoal in vocabulary.

3) *Flip cards.*

Small cards, each with one printed word from the vocabulary, colorcoded and organized in categories on a notebook ring have proved helpful. The patient quickly becomes adept in finding the appropriate card and using it to supplement his speech intelligibility. This flip-card ring prevents many frustrations in his early speech efforts. It encourages the patient to attempt conversation in his life situations rather than resorting to total writing. A card can be used to introduce and identify a new topic of conversation or a change of subjects. This technique also demonstrates that a fairly limited vocabulary can provide extensive communication, when the vocabulary is wisely chosen. This device has proved highly motivational.

4) *Gestural cues.*

In addition to the cues provided to the listener by the flip-card approach, the patient at this point can profit by some training in providing other cues and clues to his listener. An expressive gesture clarifies an otherwise unintelligible sentence. If consistency is developed in the gestures, two-way communication improves. The patient acquires swiftness of choice, ease of use, precision of sign. The persons in his daily environment find him increasingly understandable. The manual language of the deaf has many signs that may be incorporated in such a personal gestural language.

5) *Amerind Sign.*

The American Indian Sign may be a preferable choice, since it is primarily an idea-signaling system, rather than a language. Hence, the observer usually does not need formal instruction. Patients appear to acquire a fair vocabulary in it with little or no difficulty. Most of them find it amusing to do so. Its introduction at this point may provide a very welcome break in the con-

VOCAL PARAMETER MANIPULATION

I. Rate.
  A. Variation (in syllables per second).
    1. Range.
      a. Maximum.
      b. Minimum.
    2. Mean.
  B. Pauses (in a specific sample size).
    1. Incidence.
      a. Maximum.
      b. Minimum.
      c. Mean.
    2. Length.
      a. Maximum.
      b. Minimum.
      c. Mean.
  C. Vowel length.
    1. Normal + or −.
    2. Therapeutic shift.
      a. Clipping.
      b. Prolongation.
      c. Variation.

(I in relation to breath control { timing, pressure)

II. Pitch.
  A. Habitual range.
    1. Hyper ⎫
    2. Hypo ⎬ to normal.
    3. Mono ⎭
  B. Possible range.
    1. High.
    2. Low.
  C. Control.
    1. Glide.
      a. Up.
      b. Down.
    2. Breaks.
    3. Quaver.
  D. Therapeutic shifts.

III. Intensity.
  A. Range.
    1. Hyper ⎫
    2. Hypo ⎬ normal.
    3. Mono ⎭
  B. Mean (habitual).
  C. Therapeutic shifts.

IV. Quality
  A. Harsh ⎫ elimination of undesirable.
    1. Strident ⎪ modification of excessive.
  B. Nasal ⎬ manipulation of useful.
  C. Aspirate ⎭
  D. Hoarse—physician should be consulted before any therapeutic shifts are undertaken.

centrated effort the patient has been expending on oral modification.

6) *Phonatory manipulation.*

Auditory feedback from tape recordings of the patient's attempts to vary the vocal parameters can provide an effective means toward progress. Systematic drill with single sounds, words, phrases, short sentences and short paragraphs (according to the individual patient's stage of progress) may proceed step by step through the range of possible vocal parameter manipulations. The favorable results of the individual patient may be selectively applied to improve the intelligibility level of each phoneme as it is added to his sound repertoire and of words as his vocabulary expands.

Prolongation of vowels, upward shift of habitual pitch range, modification of speaking rate and control of pauses have been found most profitable. However, enough differences have appeared in individuals to make it advisable to explore all possible modifications before selecting specific vocal parameter changes for therapeutic emphasis in each case. The range of possibilities for parameter manipulation in many directions and combinations is listed in the following summary outline. It is appropriate to use this approach on the vowel and non-glossal consonants and their resulting words at this time to bring the patient's intelligibility score to its highest possible level before undertaking the glossal compensations. Phonatory manipulation may, of course, be applied to the glossal sounds and words also after they have been mastered.

b. *Glossal sounds—normal and compensatory.*

Clinical experience to the present indicates that compensations for the glossal sounds have been most quickly and successfully added to the patient's sound repertoire in the following order: [d—t], [z—s], [n], [g—k], [l], [r], [ŋ], [ð] and [θ]. The [l] and [r] indicated are the consonantal variants. These are included because some constriction or interruption of the airstream appears basic to their identification, at least in the speech of the intelligible glossectomee to date. The vowel relationships and classifications assigned to variants of these phonemes by phonetic experts are in no way ignored by this selectivity. However, they have not appeared to present critical problems in the intelligibility of the glossectomee patients so far.

With the glossal surd-sonant cognate pairs, the successful glossectomee speaker has usually achieved the sonant more easily and quickly than the cognate surd. However, after adequate development of the sonant, the surd usually appeared in the patient's repertoire spontaneously. If not, it was acquired with less drill than the sonant required. A reverse order in drill was not as productive.

    1) [d–t].

       a) *Normal production.*

       These sounds are ordinarily produced by placing the tongue tip against the alveolar ridge. Some speakers use the upper teeth rather than the gum ridge. The oral air pressure characteristic of plosives is accomplished by first closing the velopharyngeal valve, then blocking air escape with the tip of the tongue against the upper gum ridge. There is also usually a slight lowering of the mandible. Normally a complicated elevation of the tongue is involved in the air blocking. The air pressure cavity is formed between the tongue and the roof of the mouth with little or no pressure

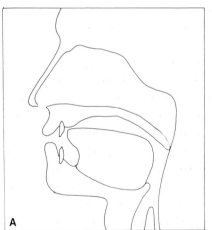 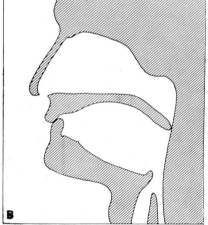

Figure 9. A, Normal tongue placement for [d] and [t]. B, Compensatory lip placement for [d] and [t].

on the cheeks. Release is accomplished by dropping the tip of the tongue.

b) *Compensatory production.*

The lower lip is used as a substitute for the tongue tip and is placed against the inner surface of the upper alveolar ridge (or teeth if present). Oral air pressure is contained by pressing the elevated lower lip firmly against the upper alveolar ridge. No lowering of the mandible is possible. This alteration of the normal appears to have little or no effect on the acoustic result. The upper lip is slightly everted. Release is accomplished by swift movement of the lower lip forward and slightly downward.

This appears to be the easiest of the compensatory synergies for the glossectomee to acquire. An immediate considerable gain in intelligibility results when initial instruction on this compensation is followed by adequate drill on [t] in all possible CV, VC, CVC and VCV combinations with each of the patient's discrete vowels. This intelligibility gain is enhanced if a prior unit has encouraged the patient to eliminate [d] and [t] as substitutes for other difficult sounds. With consistency in use of only one substitution for each difficult sound and addition of a clear [d] and [t], the patient's speech becomes much easier for the average listener to understand. Thus, there is early desirable reinforcement for the patient for his efforts.

In each instance, after the early VC, CV, VCV and CVC combinations have served their ballistic purpose, they should be eliminated and practice material confined to meaningful and useful words. A short list which avoids all glossals not yet compensated provides the most profitable drill. These may be chosen to suit each case from the materials in the appendix.

2) [z–s].

a) *Normal production.*

The [z] and [s] are classed as alveolar fricatives. The velopharyngeal valve is closed and a narrow jet of air

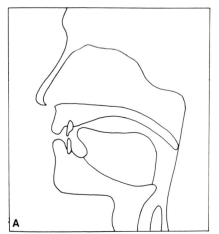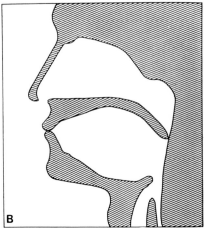

Figure 10. A, Normal tongue placement for [z] and [s]. B, Compensatory lip placement for [z] and [s].

is directed down the grooved tongue across the cutting edge of the teeth. The tongue is considered the primary agent, since the grooving is regarded as the most important positional aspect of adequate production. Successful phonemic formation is usually considered to be quite dependent on the close relationship of the upper and lower teeth. A forward and backward sliding of the mandible as well as slight eversion of the lower lip may contribute to the total result. No pressure is exerted on the cheek muscles as the air pressure cavity is contained between the tongue and the roof of the mouth.

In an alternative position for these phonemes, the tip of the tongue is low, behind the front incisors. The blade is humped and the air passes out over the grooved hump rather than the tip.

b) *Compensatory production.*

Some glossectomees have adequate upper dentures. In this case, for the compensatory [z] or [s], the air jet may be driven through a very narrow, slitlike opening between upper teeth and lower lip. In the com-

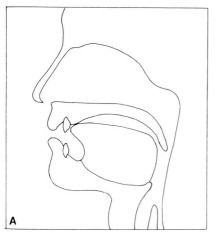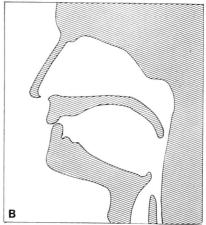

Figure 11. A, Normal tongue placement for [n]. B, Compensatory lip placement for [n].

pletely edentulous patient, both lips are tensed to create the narrow horizontal slit for air escape. Cheek compression drives the jet most effectively. In early therapy, some patients appear to use the abdominal muscles, but this is very effortful for the most of them and consequently tiring and inefficient. Drill on use of the cheek muscles is very profitable. The more intelligible speakers also slide the mandible forward slightly, causing some upward direction of the air flow. The most effective friction appears to be over the upper lip. Some slight eversion of the lower lip occurs in this case.

3) [n].

a) *Normal production.*

The [n] is described as a voiced alveolar nasal continuant. The velopharyngeal valve is open and the vocalized airstream escapes through the nose. The acoustic effect differentiating the [n] appears to be the resonance of the small oral cavity created between the tongue and the hard palate as the tongue is pressed firmly against the upper alveolar ridge. The lips are ordinarily open during the production of [n] but actually their position has little effect on the acoustic product.

b) *Compensatory production.*

The oral cavity is blocked by the lower lip touching the upper alveolar ridge. The early acoustic result is usually not adequately differentiated from the bilabial [m]. The [n] requires a more difficult adjustment than the [d−t] and [z−s] compensations. The patients whose lips are impaired have a greater problem than those who retain labial flexibility. However, consistent persistent exercising has frequently resulted in adequate increase in labial movement. The patient and clinician both need to be prepared to accept slower progress on [n] than on the prior two compensations. They must also realize that initial results will not be as satisfactory. This compensation does not stabilize or integrate as easily or as quickly as the [d−t] and [z−s]. The patient will require an increase in encouragement and support for reassurance, if he is to persist.

The clinician may wish to experiment with a labioalveolar [n] prior to the session with the patient. The positioning of the lower lip high against the inner surface of the upper alveolar ridge can produce a significantly smaller oral cavity than that present on bilabial occlusion. This difference can assist the glossectomee to contrast his [n] and [m]. The patient usually has no difficulty producing an easily recognizable [m]. Repeated drill alternating [m] and [n] will assist him to achieve more and more recognizable differentiation if he concentrates on the greatest possible reduction in oral cavity size on the [n].

Early efforts to contrast oral cavity size usually result in undesirable facial contortions. These will disappear as further practice produces expertise in finer adjustment and the patient learns exactly how much cavity size difference is required to keep his [n] within phonemic limits.

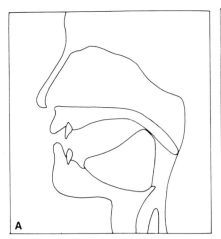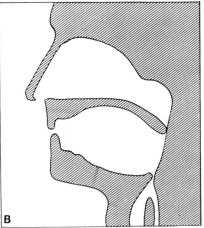

Figure 12. A, Normal tongue placement for [g] and [k]. B, Compensatory posterior pharyngeal bulge.

4) [g—k].

   a) *Normal production.*

The velopharyngeal valve is closed. Air pressure is built up and blocked from escape by the back of the tongue in contact with the soft palate. The mandible is lowered slightly. The lips are open and very slightly everted. The impounded air is released by lowering the elevated portion of the tongue without any movement of the mandible.

   b) *Compensatory production.*

The sound ceases to be linguavelar. Air pressure is blocked instead by pharyngeal constriction. Release is obtained by relaxing the stricture. The acoustic result is not a true English phoneme but resembles the glottal catch. The latter is usually heard by the listener as a moist sucking sound produced by wet adhering tissues on separation. The most intelligible glossectomee speakers have succeeded in controlling this somewhat unpleasant component, either by reducing it extensively or eliminating it entirely. This result in most cases was achieved by rigorous practice in shortening the period of stricture.

Those who failed to modify this aspect of the glottal substitution continued to have problems in differentiating the surd and sonant with ensuing confusion of [g] and [k]. However, this seldom resulted in any serious communication difficulty when all the other compensations were adequately developed.

5) [l].

a) *Normal production.*

Whether in its vowel or glide form, the [l] is usually produced by placing the tip of the tongue lightly against the upper gum ridge or the posterior surface of the upper incisors. The jaw is slightly dropped and the lips slightly open. The posterior portion of the tongue is not in lateral contact with the teeth or alveolar ridge. The airstream is thus divided, producing the only true lateral sound in English. The velopharyngeal port is closed, of course.

A dark or back [l] also appears in the sound repertoire of most normal speakers. For it, the tongue is retracted posteriorly and is humped superiorly much more than for the frontal light [l]. The airstream is divided by the posterior tongue elevation. The difference may be summarized by stating that for clear frontal [l], the forepart of the tongue approaches the hard palate, for dark posterior [l] the back part of the tongue approaches the soft palate.

b) *Compensatory production.*

Early attempts to utilize the lips as a substitute for the tongue tip in frontal [l] were completely unsuccessful with all the total glossectomee patients. Additional early experimental attempts to produce an adequate frontal [l] were all abortive. Attempts at the dark [l] were more successful.

Those patients who retained the full use of the soft palate appeared to effect the airstream division usually provided by the tongue by means of a slight vibration of the uvula subtly apparent in the cinefluorograms. Patients with altered soft palate or without

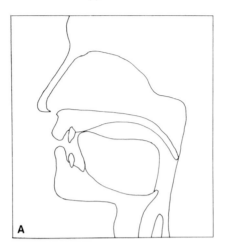

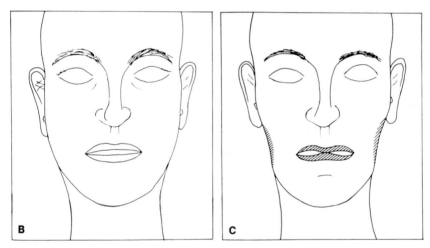

Figure 13. A, Normal tongue placement for [l]. The diagram does not show the lateral escape of air regarded as necessary to adequate phoneme production. B, Normal lip position for [l]. The lips can be abducted to a greater degree within phonemic limits. C, Compensatory lip and cheek position for [l].

adequate control of the remaining uvula seemed to achieve the dark [l] by means of buccal constriction. The cheeks appear to be drawn inward and to vibrate slightly. The acoustic result is not as satisfactory but is identifiable, although distorted.

Even the clearest uvular [l] continues to be slightly distorted, even for the most successful speakers.

Very recently, a successful front [l] has evolved from further labial efforts. The successful speakers make the air division with the lips lightly touching in the center and open toward both left and right lip corners. Some patients report that they profited by the attempts to differentiate [l] and [r] and consequently improved both.

6) [r].

a) *Normal production.*

To produce consonantal [r], a resonating cavity of unusual shape appears necessary. The posterior portion of the tongue must be elevated but also some of the anterior tongue elevated still further. In many instances, the tip serves this function, in others the tongue blade. The point of the tongue, wide and thin, is slightly retroflexed, forming a small hollow just behind the tip. The velopharyngeal valve is closed. The airstream is directed over the upturned tongue tip and is prevented from escaping over the lateral edges into the buccal cavity. The tip of the tongue is in vibration. The tongue does not touch the roof of the mouth. The [r] is a postalveolar linguapalatal voiced continuous glide, sometimes classified as a liquid.

Although two frequently occurring tongue positions are usually described, actually this phoneme is the least stabile and describable of the English list. There is no static position identifiable for it. Rather, it is the product of a sequence of movements creating a rapid change of resonance.

b) *Compensatory production.*

Glossectomee speakers who achieve any serviceable intelligibility level appear to have little difficulty with the vowel forms [ɜ] and [ɝ]. In early consonant drill, they substitute these for the consonantal [r] and later under instruction shift to [w] as the substitution.

Those who produce an adequate consonantal [r]

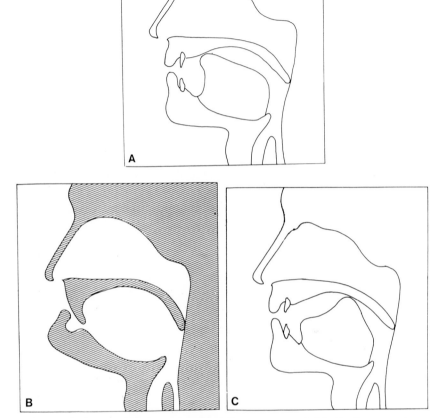

Figure 14. A, Normal tongue position for consonantal [r]. B, Compensatory lip position. C, Normal tongue position alternative for [r].

seem to create the resonating cavity of the required unusual shape by means of a combination of buccal compression and anterior mandibular thrust. Phonetic descriptions of the unusual shape for normal speech vary but include a relationship among a small anterior resonating cavity connecting with a larger posterior cavity by a narrow, funnellike channel. Some of the successful glossectomee speakers achieve this as a result of the mandibular thrust by retroverting the lower lip. The upper lip thus divides the oral space into a large buccal cavity (with a narrow channel under the upper lip) and a smaller anterior cavity just inside the lower retroverted lip. Where this has been accomplished, the speaker's [r] is rather close to the normal acoustic effect. Of all the glossal phonemes, [r] has the greatest variation and least stability for glossectomees, as for normals.

Many patients who fail to achieve buccal control and the associated lip compensation have managed an identifiable [r] by a substitute pharyngeal grunt-like resonance. A number of these have improved this sound by drills which combine a short energetic grunt with the lip shape for [w]. In a series of repetitions, they slowly modify the lip rounding into lip flattening. In this fashion, the acoustic result has been slowly shifted from a distinct [w] to a sound resembling [r] at the lower extreme of its phonemic limits. With continued drill, the sound becomes more and more acceptable. A few of these with patience and persistence have finally managed the lip relationships for the most satisfactory compensation.

7) [ŋ].
 a) *Normal production.*

The velopharyngeal valve is open and the vocalized airstream escapes through the nose. The oral cavity is blocked by the posterior humping of the tongue into firm contact with the velum at its attachment to the hard palate.

 b) *Compensatory production.*

Adequacy for [ŋ] compensation is highly related to the patient's prior success with [n] and [g]. When both have been adequately achieved, the patient's [n] is modified into [ŋ] by addition of the glottal. In the earliest attempts to determine an order of difficulty for the glossal sounds, the [ŋ] was first placed immediately following the [n]. Later it was postponed

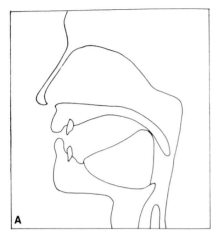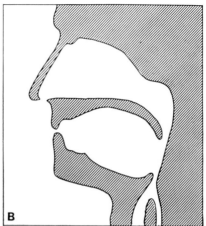

Figure 15. A, Normal tongue position for [ŋ]. B, Compensatory posterior pharyngeal bulge.

to follow [g—k]. It now appears that neither of these placements is optimal. Both seemed to interfere with adequate differentiation of [l] and [r] for reasons as yet undetermined.

Patients with a less than adequate [n] substitute the glottal alone for the [ŋ]. However, some small nasal resonance appears on the spectrograms, so probably they are really combining the barely adequate [n] with the glottal. Provided all the other glossal sounds have been clearly differentiated, this glottal substitution, if consistent, does not seriously affect intelligibility after the listener has identified the substitution.

8) [ð—θ].

a) *Normal production.*

These phonemes result from placing the tip of the tongue almost in contact with the posterior surface of the upper incisors or with their cutting edge. The air built up by velopharyngeal closure is thus directed between the tongue and teeth in a broad stream of minimal height. This opening will vary individually. The mandible must be delicately balanced so that the lower teeth do not bite the tongue but are merely

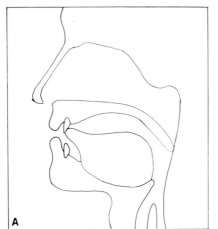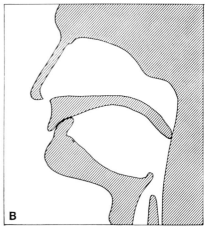

Figure 16. A, Normal tongue position for [ð] and [θ]. B, Compensatory lip position for [ð] and [θ].

touching it lightly to steady it. Some speakers extend the tongue tip between the upper and lower incisors. There is some eversion of the lips and usually no pressure on the cheeks.

b) *Compensatory production.*

Compensation for these phonemes has proved the most difficult task in glossectomee therapy. Development of a usable compensation has occurred only recently and as yet only a few speakers have mastered it.

Patients with the upper central incisors intact or with an adequate upper denture place the lower lip inside the upper teeth, building up air pressure, then releasing it in a short energetic burst by drawing the lower lip down and forward against the teeth. Early attempts resembled [d–t]. Persistent drill on shortening and energizing the release tends to improve the result.

A few edentulous patients are managing the sound with the lower lip placed slightly inside the upper lip and then moved forward and downward against it quickly for the release. Persistent explorations of varying modification of the exact contact and the release speed have improved the acoustic result in every case, although to varying degrees. A slight improvement resulting in even minimal differentiation between [ð–θ] and [d–t] has considerable impact on the intelligibility score.

9) *Phonatory manipulation.*

(See a. 6 under nonglossal consonants and apply to glossals.)

10) *Glossal summary.*

   a) Instruct the patient in the compensatory pattern.

   b) Have him attempt to produce it in all possible combinations with his discrete vowels, with goal of

      (1) Adequate auditory discrimination and self-monitoring.

      (2) Kinetic control and monitoring through

         (a) Conscious physiologic adjustment.

         (b) Reliable replication.

   c) Combine with the non-glossal consonants and extract words for daily useful vocabulary.

   d) Combine with remaining vowels in the vowel triangle for the same purpose.

   e) Manipulate pitch and vowel duration with word list.

   f) Develop short sentences and add rate manipulation.

   g) Combine several short sentences and add pause manipulation, also directives in Chapter VI.

   h) Arrange available vocabulary by categories for life situations: job, money, market, bank, post office, drug store, travel, department store, directions, family, friends, conversation on sports on television, discussion of weather, politics or recent news. Assign one for use and a report on success or failure.

   c. *Consonant Review.*

At this point, a systematic examination of the patient's phonemic products for analysis of his remaining problems is pertinent. The latter may then be arranged in order of difficulty for review and further drill. By continuing efforts to perfect the least troublesome of the residual deficiencies, and by complementing this with a consistent substitution pattern the patient will achieve and continue to improve useful daily life communication.

Chapter X

CONCLUSION

SPECIAL CONSIDERATIONS FOR PARTIAL
GLOSSECTOMEES

THE PATIENT with partial excision of the tongue may not require as much (or even any) of the vowel, non-glossal and glossal consonant drill as the total glossectomee. His speech rehabilitation plan possibly may be approached as an articulation problem and treated as such. If his hearing is intact (or at least serviceable for speech discrimination), he may need only articulation assistance on a few deviant phonemes.

The rehabilitation plan for this patient will, of course, be individual, as usual, and depend on the assessment of his present deficiencies, his preoperative articulation level, dialects, education, job, age, family, motivation and any special needs. He probably can achieve the glossal sounds with considerably less physiologic compensation than that needed by the patient with total excision.

His target goal in intelligibility may well coincide with his preoperative speech. A number of these patients have even improved beyond their preoperative level as a result of the improved auditory discrimination and kinetic feedback developed in the speech clinic. The final result may depend on the amount and locus of the excision and the flexibility of the residual tongue.

If the excision is limited to the tongue tip, there may be only minor initial distortion in sounds related specifically to tongue tip precision. The larger the segment, the greater the distortion which seems to appreciate not linearly but logarithmically. Some patients with a large anterior portion of the tongue removed do not achieve as high an intelligibility score as a number of the total glossectomees. Pitch elevation has improved some scores considerably.

When the surgery involves only a lateral segment and the residual tongue is flexible, prognosis for quick restoration of intelligibility is very favorable.

In admission evaluation, the partial glossectomee should have special attention in testing his physiologic competence to provide adequate normal obstruction within normal locus limits. He may be able to use the residual tongue for one or even many of the glossal sounds. His divergence from the normal sound patterns may be so slight that treatment is not needed or warranted. He may, on the other hand, need compensations for one or more of the glossal sounds. Occasionally a partial glossectomee requires the same detailed rehabilitation procedures planned for those with total excision.

LARYNGECTOMEES

Five laryngectomees who are also total glossectomees have been included in the project to date. Two of them have achieved minimal communication through use of the glossectomee compensations applied to a reed larynx. The electronic larynx did not serve the purpose, as its vibration pattern obscured the adaptive articulation.

Two others who do not have sufficient oral flexibility as yet for instrument-speech attempts to be profitable are using the flip cards mentioned earlier. Two are experimenting with Indian Sign Language and are achieving gratifying success with this approach in communication. One has interspersed the signs with some finger spelling when the occasion requires. All of these approaches provide faster communication than writing.

THE FUTURE

Discussion to this point has dealt with the problem of tongue cancer, total glossectomy and speech rehabilitation, the history of the latter and clinical treatment and research to date. In addition to historical perspective on the past and report on the present, it is necessary for progress to look forward.

Many discussions have developed from the publications and

workshops. Numerous clinicians are now involved in speech rehabilitation of glossectomees previously not referred for treatment. Research personnel are undertaking further exploration of the total problem and various aspects not yet considered. Results from both clinic and research will hopefully enlarge and enhance the work presented here. It is possible it will change and negate it by discovering different and better ways to serve these patients. These will be joyfully welcomed, as such service is the ultimate purpose of this volume and its contributors.

BIBLIOGRAPHY

American Cancer Society: *Maintenance of Oral and General Health in the Management of the Oral Cancer Patient.* New York, American Cancer Society, 1968, 1969.

American Cancer Society: *Cancer Facts and Figures.* New York, American Cancer Society, 1969, 1972.

Arnold, G. E.: Speech without a Tongue. In Luchsinger, R., and Arnold, G. E.: *Clinical Communicology.* Belmont, Wadsworth, 1965, pp. 656–657.

Backus, O. L.: Speech rehabilitation following excision of the tip of the tongue. *American Journal of the Disabled Child, 60:*368–370, 1940.

Bloomer, H. H.: Observations on palatopharyngeal movement in speech and deglutition. *Journal of Speech and Hearing Disorders, 18:*230–246, 1953.

Boone, D.: *The Voice and Voice Therapy.* Englewood Cliffs, Prentice-Hall, 1971.

Brodnitz, F. S.: Speech after glossectomy. *Current Problems in Phoniatrics and Logopedics.* Basel, Karger, 1960.

Brodnitz, F. S.: *Vocal Rehabilitation.* Rochester, American Academy of Ophthalmology, 1965.

C.I.D.: *Auditory Test W-22.* St. Louis, Central Institute for the Deaf, 1952.

Davis, H. and Silverman, R.: *Hearing and Deafness,* 3rd ed. New York, Holt, 1970.

Dillenschneider, E., Broustet, M., Levy, D., and Greiner, G.: Place de sonographie dans une consultation de phoniatre. *Journal Functional Otorhinolaryngologie, 18:*383–386, 1969.

Donaldson, R. C., Skelly, M., and Paletta, F. X.: Total glossectomy for cancer. *American Journal of Surgery, 116:*585–590, 1968.

Eskew, H. A., and Shepard, E. E.: Congenital aglossia. *American Journal of Orthodontics, 35:*116–119, 1949.

Fletcher, S. G.: Processes and maturation of mastication and deglutition. *Speech and the Dentofacial Complex, ASHA Reports No. 5.* Washington, American Speech and Hearing Association, 1970, pp. 92–105.

French, N., and Steinberg, G.: Factors governing intelligibility of speech sounds. *Journal of the Acoustical Society of America, 19,* 1947.

Froeschels, E.: *Lehrbuch der Sprachheilkunde,* 3rd ed. Wien, Deuticke, 1931.

Froeschels, E.: *Speech Therapy.* Boston, Expression, 1931.

Froeschels, E., Kastein, S., and Weiss, D.: A method of therapy for paralytic conditions of the mechanisms of phonation, respiration and glutination. *Journal of Speech and Hearing Disorders, 20:* 365–370, 1955.

Frowen, V. K., and Moser, H.: Relation of dentition to speech. *Journal of the American Dental Association, 31:*1801–1090, 1944.

Garliner, D.: The speech therapist's role in myo-functional therapy. *New York State Dental Journal, 32:*169–172, 1966.

Glemser, Bernard: *Man Against Cancer.* New York, Funk and Wagnalls, 1969.

Goldstein, M.: Speech without a tongue. *Journal of Speech Disorders, 5:*65–69, 1940.

Goldstein, M.: New concepts of the function of the tongue. *Laryngoscope, 50:*164–188, 1940.

Greene, J. S.: Anomalies of the speech mechanism and associated voice and speech disorders. *New York Journal of Medicine, 45:* 605–608, 1945.

Gutzmann, H.: Der Zuzammenhang von Sprache in du Geschichte der Medizin. *Manuskriptchronik du Geschichte du Sprachheilk, 12:* 289, 1902.

Herberman, M. A.: Rehabilitation of patients following glossectomy. *Archives of Otolaryngology, 67:*182–183, 1958.

Hoops, R. A.: *Speech Science: Acoustics in Speech.* Springfield, Thomas, 1969.

House, A. S.: Formant band-width and vowel preference. *Journal of Speech and Hearing Research, 3:*1–5, 1960.

Keaster, J.: Studies in the anatomy and physiology of the tongue. *Laryngoscope, 50:*222–257, 1940.

Kremer, A.: Cancer of the tongue. *Minnesota Medicine, 36:*828–830, 1953.

Kussmaul, A.: *Die Störungen der Sprache.* Leipzig, Vogel, 1910.

Martin, H. E.: History of lingual cancer. *American Journal of Surgery, 48:*703–716, 1940.

Martin, H. E., Munster, H., and Sugarbaker, E.: Cancer of the tongue. *Archives of Surgery, 41:*888–936, 1940.

Massengill, R., Jr.; Maxwell, S., and Pickrell, K.: Swallowing characteristics noted in a glossectomy patient. *Plastic Reconstructive Surgery, 45:*89–91, 1970.

Massengill, R., Jr., Maxwell, S., and Pickrell, K.: An analysis of articulation following partial and total glossectomy. *Journal of Speech and Hearing Disorders, 35:*170–173, 1970.

McDonald, E. T.: *Articulation Testing and Treatment.* Pittsburgh, Stanwix House, 1965.

McEnerny, E. T., and Gaines, F. P.: Tongue tie in infants and children. *Journal of Pediatrics, 18:*252–255, 1941.

McQuarrie, D.: Immediate functional restoration of the mandible after surgical treatment of advanced oral cancer. *Archives of Surgery, 102:*447–449, 1971.

Panconcelli-Calzia, G.: Uber die Wiedererlangung der Sprechfahigheit nach Zingenverletzun. *Deutche Millitar Arzt, 8:*270, 1943.

Pare, A.: *Chirurgion Workes.* London, 1634.

Perkell, J. S.: *Physiology of Speech Production.* Cambridge, M.I.T., 1969.

Perkins, W.: Vocal function: assessment and therapy. In Travis, L. (Ed.) : *Handbook of Speech Pathology and Audiology.* New York, Appleton-Century, 1971.

Sheldon, R. L., Jr.: Therapeutic exercise and speech pathology. *ASHA,* 855–859, 1963.

Sheldon, R. L., Jr., Brooks, A., and Youngstrom, K.: Articulation and patterns of palatopharyngeal closure. *Journal of Speech and Hearing Disorders, 29:*390–408, 1964.

Sheldon, R. L., Jr., Brooks, A., and Youngstron, K.: Clinical assessment of palatopharyngeal closure. *Journal of Speech and Hearing Disorders, 30:*37–43, 1965.

Skelly, M., Spector, D., Donaldson, R., Brodeur, A., and Paletta, F.: Compensatory physiologic phonetics for the glossectomee. *Journal of Speech and Hearing Disorders, 36:*101–114, 1971a.

Skelly, M., Donaldson, R., Scheer, G., and Guzzardo, M.: Dysphonias associated with spinal bracing in scoliosis. *Journal of Speech and Hearing Disorders, 36:*368–376, 1971b.

Skelly, M., and Donaldson, R.: Glossectomee Speech Rehabilitation Procedures. In *Proceedings of the XV Congress of Logopedics and Phoniatrics.* Buenos Aires, Ares, 1972a.

Skelly, M., Donaldson, R., Fust, R., and Townsend, D.: Changes in Phonatory Aspects of Glossectomee Intelligibility Through Vocal Parameter Manipulation. *Journal of Speech and Hearing Disorders, 37,* Nov., 1972b.

Subtelny, J.: Examination of current philosophies associated with swallowing behavior. *American Journal of Orthodontics, 51:*161–182, 1965.

Thomas, I. B.: Influence of first and second formants on the intelligibility of speech. *Journal of the Audio Engineering Society, 16:* 182–185, 1968.

Thomas, I. B.: Perceived pitch of whispered vowels. *Journal of the Acoustical Society of America, 46:*468–470. 1969.

Travis, L.: *Handbook of Speech Pathology.* New York, Appleton-Century, 1957.

Trible, W. M.: The rehabilitation of deglutition following head and neck surgery. *Laryngoscope,* 518–523, 1967.

Twistleton, E. *The Tongue Not Essential to Speech.* London, John Murray, 1873.

Weinberg, B.: Deglutition: a review of selected topics. *Speech and the Dentofacial Complex.* ASHA Reports No. 5: 116–131, 1970. Washington, American Speech and Hearing Association, 1970.

Zimmerman, J. D.: Speech Production after Glossectomy. Unpublished paper, American Speech and Hearing Association Convention, 1958.

APPENDIX

RESEARCH-RELATED MATERIALS

GLOSSAL MONOSYLLABLE LIST

1. they	11. nay	21. say	31. lay	41. day
2. go	12. rue	22. or	32. your	42. ear
3. eel	13. add	23. lea	33. an	43. all
4. no	14. though	24. row	34. do	44. knee
5. sue	15. on	25. saw	35. as	45. so
6. ray	16. deed	26. gay	36. ran	46. that
7. dough	17. are	27. owed	37. low	47. dad
8. thew	18. ooze	28. thee	38. new	48. ease
9. oath	19. thaw	29. see	39. awed	49. youth
10. goo	20. air	30. aid	40. through	50. ale

GLOSSECTOMY FUNCTIONAL COMMUNICATION
LIST #1

1. What is your last name?
2. Spell it, please.
3. First name?
4. Middle initial, if any?
5. In what state do you live?
6. City?
7. Street?
8. House number?
9. What is your social security number?
10. In what year were you born?
11. What month?
12. What date?
13. How old are you?
14. Are you married?
15. Your children's names? (If none, substitute a parental first name or that of a wife.)
16. Who is your next of kin?
17. How long have you been sick?
18. Have you been in the hospital here?
19. When? (Or what other hospital were you in?)
20. What ward? (Or who was your doctor at home?)

145

21. Do you have an appointment today?
22. Who is your doctor here at the V.A.?
23. When was your last appointment?
24. How did you get here today?
25. What is the weather like outside today?

GLOSSECTOMY FUNCTIONAL COMMUNICATION
LIST #2

1. What year is this?
2. What month is this?
3. What day of the week is this?
4. What's the date?
5. What time is it?
6. Have you an appointment at the Speech Clinic?
7. Who is your clinician (in the Speech Clinic) ?
8. Where is the Speech Clinic?
9. When did you eat last? (lunch, breakfast)
10. What did you have for (lunch, breakfast) ?
11. Are you working or retired?
12. What kind of work do (did) you do?
13. What branch of the service were you in?
14. What war?
15. Where did you serve?
16. What are your hobbies?
17. What's your favorite sport?
18. What program do you like on TV?
19. Which newspaper do you read?
20. What's your favorite magazine?
21. Do you buy anything in the Canteen?
22. Do you smoke now? Ever smoke?
23. Are you taking any medicine now?
24. Have you had any immunizations in the last six months? (shots)
25. Anyone in family ill in the last six months?

TEST MATERIALS

PATIENT HISTORY, BACKGROUND AND TASTES

Name: Date: Time:
Address: Hosp. No.:
Phone: Ward: Outpatient:
Birthdate: Physician:
Family contact: Surgery date:
Address: ASP Examiner:
Phone: Hosp. address:
Relationship:

Brief medical history related to current problem:
Principal health problems:
Describe any use of:
   Tobacco
   Alcohol
   Snuff
Describe current eating procedures and problems:
Describe any swallowing problems:
Describe education briefly:
Employment:
Future plans or hopes:
Responsibilities to his family:
Attitudes affecting rehabilitation:
Intelligence level: (examiner's opinion)
Attach Leiter scores and records and any Psychology and Social
   Service reports.
   Gregarious or a loner:
   Talker or a listener:
   Like large party or a few friends:
   Talk: Drink: Play loud games: Loud music:
   Play silent games: Watch TV: Listen Hi-fi:
   Read: Draw: Paint: Play musical instrument:
   Work with tools: Garden: Travel:
   Favorite sport:

Favorite music:
Favorite reading:
Favorite hobby:

MEDICAL AND SURGICAL DATA

Name: *Hosp. No.*   *Date:*

Surgery	*Intact*	*Excised*	*Total*	*Partial*	*Right*	*Left*	*Bilateral*	*Superior*	*Inferior*	*Anterior*	*Posterior*
Tongue											
Mandible											
Maxilla											
Labia											
Teeth											
Gingiva											
Palate											
Velum											
Uvula											
Epiglottis											
Floor of mouth											
Neck											

Stages:
Cobalt:

Nerves	*Intact*	*Impaired*	*Notes*
Vagus			
Sup. laryngeal			
Thyrohyoid			
Hypoglossal			
Inf. constrictor			

Cervical sympathetic
Phrenic
Brachial plexus
Muscles
Labial
Mandibular
Velar
Buccal

Dysphagia:
CNS problems:
Visual:
Auditory:
Tactual:
Diadochokinetic rate:

Attach Audiogram and any consult report.

GLOSSECTOMEE SPEECH EVALUATION

(Record patient on 5-inch tape under standard conditions; include clinician voice asking questions.)

A. Questions.
  1. What is your full name?
  2. Where do you live (number, street, city, state, zip) ?
  3. Tell me about your trip to the hospital.
  4. Who is your doctor?
  5. What is the weather like outside today?

B. Reading.
Have patient read *Arthur the Rat*. (If he is unintelligible, stop as soon as you have made this judgment.)

C. Abbreviated phonetic inventory.
  1. Nonglossal consonants and vowels (record patient saying) :
    Why buy ham?
    May we have pie?
    You owe me a fee.
  2. Glossal consonants and vowels:
    I am giving her the little red coats for Nora.
  3. Aspirate effect:
    Helen hollers "Hi, Harry, hurry home."

D. Phonation.

    Instruct patient as follows:

    1. Say the word "high" on the highest note you can reach.

    2. Say the word "low" on your lowest note.

    3. Go from your lowest note to your highest on "hello." (glide)

    4. Go from your highest to your lowest on "Hello."

    5. Judge range,   up glide range,   down glide range.

        Normal (octave) :   Normal: Normal:

        More: Interrupted: Interrupted:

        Less: Impossible: Impossible:

Instruct patient to take one ordinary breath, then make the sound you indicate, making the sound last as long as the breath does. Have him practice it once before recording and timing the three trials on each sound. Use stopwatch.

    6. Surd [f]:   sec.   sec.   sec.

    7. Sonant [v]:   sec.   sec.   sec.

    8. Resonant [a]:   sec.   sec.   sec.

Record and time one trial on each of the vowels:

    9. [e]:   sec.

    10. [i]:   sec.

    11. [aɪ]:   sec.

    12. [o]:   sec.

    13. [u]:   sec.

E. Patient evaluation of clearest and easiest vowel.

    14. Which does he think is clearest and best?

    15. Which can he make most easily?

F. Glossal consonants with vowel [o], each timed three times. (Clinician should not record his own production. Explain that item 17 is a girl's name) .

    16. dough

    17. Zoe

    18. no

    19. go

    20. low

    21. row

    22. though

    23. ping pong

G. Nonglossal words (items 25 through 34).
Choose at random one of the groups of ten from the list, presenting printed cards in random order:

beep	boy	babe	buy	bay
five	Fay	foam	fame	fee
hay	high	he	Hugh	ham
my	maam	map	may	mom
pope	pipe	pay	pop	pave
Vi	view	vim	veep	via
wave	we	why	wipe	wife
yap	yoyo	yippee	yeh	yup
bum	beam	buoy	beef	bib
owe	eve	ape	aim	heap

Three listeners score the tape:

    a. The clinician (prognostic).
    b. The patient (goal).
    c. Untrained listener unfamiliar with patient (progress).

H. Nonglossal sentences (items 35 through 44)
Choose at random one of the sentence groups, and present printed cards in random order:

List 1

    Why buy ham?
    Have you a hoe?
    May I have a few?
    Wipe my yoyo, Fay.
    Mom, may we have pie maybe?
    You yap, I'm mum.
    Weigh my puppy.
    Papa, pay off.
    Buy a whip.
    Move my hay.

List 2

    I owe Amy a fee.
    Have you a map?
    May hope be high, Babe.
    Bob may move the heavy boom.

Byebye fame if I'm a bum.
I have beef, you have ham.
Weigh my wife.
Aim my way.
Buy me a heap.
Move my pipe.

List 3

Hop a hoop, bum.
How may I aim?
We may have a way.
Have you a highway map?
I weave a web, you weave a woof.
Abe may have a wife.
Weigh my ham.
Buy a poem.
Hoe my hay.
Move my heap, Bud.

List 4

Move my mop, Bob.
May I have five?
You owe me a fee.
Hugh may heap the hay high.
I aim at fame, I pay my way.
Wipe my bum eye, Bub.
My hope is high, Mom.
Weigh my beef.
Buy me a hoe.
Pay my wife.

List 5

Buy my pie.
Have you my hoe?
You mope, I mop.
Maybe you pave my highway?
Aim my puppy home, Mame.
Hop my heap, Pop.
Weigh my hay, Abe.
Ape my Pop, boy.

Buy a map, Babe.

Move my whip, Amy.

I. Record patient speaking each of four words (foam, wipe, heap, pave) ((items 45 through 53) under following conditions:

With greater muscular vigor (labial),

With wider jaw excursion (mandibular),

At faster speed (rate),

At slower speed (rate),

With jaw moving forward (thrust),

At higher pitch (frequency),

With vowel prolongation (duration),

With increased loudness (intensity),

With decreased loudness (intensity).

J. Total English phoneme survey.

Choose at random one of the Every Day Sentences

Lists (Davis and Silverman) and present cards in random order. (items 54 through 63).

K. Auditory memory span.

Present patient with box of ten common objects. Choose one at random and ask him to hand it to you. Return item to box each time. Increase the number, varying the objects and the order, until he fails three in succession. The last successful reply measures his word memory span for purposes of this evaluation. If span is below seven, further testing is indicated. The response level should be evaluated in relation to his audiogram.

AUDIOLOGY AND SPEECH PATHOLOGY

Leiter Report

Name: Hosp. No.   Date:

LEITER SCORE:

OBSERVATION OF PATIENT RESPONSES (Please use red ink):

Quick attack: Delayed:

Fast completion: Slow:

Corrected mistakes unassisted: Quickly:

              assisted: Slowly:

Learned by demonstration (number of trials) :
        Quickly: Slowly: Not at all:
Color cued responses are better
                poorer than black and white.
Shape cued responses are better
                poorer than picture/color.
Numerical responses are better
                poorer than non numerical.
Patient distorted responses by: With:
  Inversion: Consistently: Shape:
  Rotation: Inconsistently: Color:
                                Numbers:

Attitudes and behavior when corrected:
  Rejected: Applied: Ignored:
  Accepted: Departed:
  Ceased to respond: Became emotional:
Did patient seek clinician approval of completed task?
Was he indifferent to it?
Patient order of attack on task:
    Random order:
    Seeks stall for nearest block:
    Places blocks in order of nearness:
    Seeks block for first stall:
    Places blocks in stall order:
    Begins with middle stall:
    Begins with middle block:
    Works to right, then to left:
    Works to left, then to right:
    Alternates from middle:
    Uses visual scan to locate stall appropriate:
    Uses manual scan:
    Makes corrections in progress:
    If the last block is obviously incorrect due to prior error, describe how he proceeds to solve his problem: (use reverse side)
    Did patient request help: Demand it: Reject it:
      Always: Frequently: Occasionally: Infrequently: No:
    When error was indicated, did patient:

Perseverate in prior responses:
Make random incorrect changes:
Change one stall at a time experimentally:
Withdraw all blocks and begin again:
Withdraw incorrect blocks and place correctly:
Did fatigue appear: Gradually: Suddenly:

GLOSSECTOMEE SPEECH REHABILITATION
Tape Recording
Videocording

Name: Hosp. No.   Date:

Recording conditions: (Attach specs. if standard)
Room: Videocorder make:
Time of day: Tape Recorder make:
Ambient noise level: Microphone type:
Recording level: Distance to lips:
Non standard conditions: Standard conditions:
Explain:
Patient conditions:
Fatigued: Glasses lacking:
Sleepy: Hearing aid lacking:
Hungry: Ambulatory:
Medicated: Escorted:
Distractable: Cart:
Emotional: Other:
Materials recorded:
Reel marking and identification:
Recording technician:
Comments:

DRILL MATERIALS

CARRIER PHRASES

1. Have you a . . . ?
2. Have you my . . . ?
3. He may have a . . . .
4. He may have my . . . .
5. Why buy a . . . ?
6. I am . . . .
7. May I have a . . . ?
8. Buy me a . . . .
9. You owe me a . . . .
10. Who may have a . . . ?
11. I move a . . . .
12. I aim my . . . .
13. Be a . . . .
14. I have a . . . .
15. I may buy a . . . .
16. May I have five . . . ?
17. Move my . . . .
18. Mop my . . . .
19. Weigh my . . . .
20. Wipe my . . . .

NON-GLOSSAL WORDS

Abby	baby	boop	eye	half
Abe	bay	bop	ewe	ham
Ahab	be	bough	fame	have
aim	bee	bow	Fay	hay
am	beam	boy	fee	he
Amy	beef	bub	feif	heap
ape	beep	buff	few	heavy
away	bib	bum	fife	hem
awe	Bob	buoy	five	hew
aye	bomb	buy	foam	high
Bab	boob	bye	fop	hip
babe	boom	eve	fume	hive

hobo	map	pap	we	aim
hoe	may	papa	weave	be
home	maybe	pave	web	buy
hoop	maw	pay	weep	bow
hop	me	paw	whim	have
hope	mew	peep	whip	hew
hove	miff	pew	who	hoe
how	mime	pie	whom	hop
hub	mob	pipe	why	hope
Hugh	Mom	poem	wife	imbibe
hum	moo	pompom	wipe	imbue
hump	mop	pop	womb	mow
him	mope	pope	woe	owe
I	move	pub	woo	pay
if	movie	puff	yap	pave
imbibe	mow	puppy	yam	wave
imbue	muff	veep	yea	weave
imp	mum	via	you	weigh
Ma	my	vie	yoyo	weep
ma'am	oboe	view	Yuma	whip
Mab	of	vim	up	wipe
maim	off	wave		woo
mama	ohm	waif	*verbs*	vie
Mame	owe	way	am	vow

GLOSSAL WORDS AND SENTENCES
FOR SPECIFIC PHONEMES

[d] [t]

day	due	ate	pat	hot
aid	deb	evade	vat	pot
ate	deaf	I'd	bet	what
dame	deputy	you'd	met	add
Dave	dab	owed	pet	potato
die	daffy	bat	vet	doom
dough	dam	fat	wet	dupe
do	adapt	hat	bought	bade
dew	daub	mat	fought	fade

made	beet	bit	wide	it
paid	bead	bid	Maude	odd
wade	feed	fit	pawed	hood
bed	weed	hit	wad	wowed
fed	bad	hid	booed	mowed
wed	fad	bite	mood	abode
head	had	bide	wooed	abide
boot	mad	boat	wood	abutt
food	pad	moat	would	abate
hoot	Ed	vote	at	abbot
moot	Edie			

Today I ate a potato.
A daffy dame was my doom.
My house is wide: my house is high.
Dave paid dough; you hid the wad.
My food is too hot.

[z] [s]

say	see	his	sup	sap
ace	ease	Bess	sop	sob
base	sum	bass	miss	soft
safe	some	boss	saw	salve
face	Eve	mass	booze	mess
same	seep	pass	abuse	piece
mace	peace	moss	is	pose
save	sigh	moose	as	posy
vase	ice	muse	sift	vast
pace	mice	so	Sam	pessimist
ways	vice	sofa	sip	vamoose
muss	miss	sub	soup	

I say I saw him.
It's so easy to say so.
My ace is high, so you sigh, you buy.
Sew it as I say.
Ayes have it, so moved.

[n]

in	on	name	nave	knife
an	nay	nape	knave	nigh

no	ban	men	when	knees
new	bonnie	man	van	knives
nebby	fane	hewn	wan	nose
nab	find	immune	wind	news
knob	phone	pain	Nate	pains
bane	hen	pone	night	veins
bean	fan	pen	not	bones
bind	main	pan	net	nod
bone	mean	pawn	neat	moans
boon	mind	wound	nods	boons
been	moan	vein	napes	moons
Ben	moon	vain		

(Additional words may be created by pluralizing and by adding "ed.")

What's the main news today?

What do we have to eat tonight, a pan of beans?

Didn't you say you want a fan?

I nabbed the phone tonight but got no news.

I mean I have a pain in my knee bones.

[g] [k]

Kay	gam	comb	mock	goat
gay	gob	cope	invoke	goad
key	gop	cove	Maggie	good
guy	goof	bike	pagan	gut
go	gain	beg	vague	add
goo	came	make	fig	keyed
cuckoo	cape	wake	bag	kid
ache	cave	weak	big	Ked
aigue	cap	woke	fag	cod
game	cab	Kim	bog	cawed
gape	cafe	Kip	fog	code
gave	cam	pack	pike	cud
give	cab	back	poke	kit
gift	cop	fact	puke	Kate
gap	coup	Mack	gad	cat
gab	coffee	peek	God	
gaff	keep	meek	got	

caught	cut	baked	vacate
coat	kept	faked	hacked

Kate kept back two facts.
Kim got caught at poker.
He gave me a poke and took my coat.
I goofed on my coffee; it's no good.
My cape is big and keeps out fog.

[1]

lay	lead	loam	fool	love
lee	leaf	loom	foal	bull
lie	life	lamb	hill	fill
low	loaf	ball	mole	Hal
Lou	laugh	fall	pole	mill
Libby	bile	hole	pool	pal
lab	file	mile	leave	fell
bale	heel	pile	alive	hull
fail	meal	pull	louver	mall
hail	peel	vile	bell	pall
mail	pole	leap	full	golf
pale	veal	elope	hill	all
hale	lame	loop	hell	ill
veil	lime	lap	mule	eel
wail	loan	bill	pill	ale
vale				

Laugh a lot if you want to live well.
Loam is good for leaves.
Fill my plate, I like lamb and veal.
A hole up hill is full of golf balls.
My bills pile up in my mail.

[r]

ray	arrow	write	rot	barrow
rye	Mary	rote	rut	berry
row	merry	root	rib	Harry
array	marry	Rit	rob	raid
arrive	rate	rat	rub	ride

road	rough	rum	reap	rave
rude	ream	harrow	ripe	rove
rid	rhyme	fairy	rope	raw
rod	roam	parry	rip	borrow
reef	room	hairy	rep	very
rife	rim	rape	rap	virus
roof	ram			

He was very merry when he arrived in my room.
Are any berry bushes ripe to reap?
Harry ribbed Mary about her writing but he married her.
Our road gives a rough ride.
I wrote at a very rapid rate.

[ŋ]

bang	pingpong	wrong	ring	sing
fang	dingdong	wrung	rang	sang
hang	singsong	wring	rung	song
Ming	kingkong	king	bung	sung

(Add "ing" to all above)
His Ming vase is a long way from home.
Fong sang in a singsong tone.
The gong rang dingdong.
Pingpong is a bang up game.
His king righted a long standing wrong.

[ð] [θ]

they	thew	that	loath	them
thee	heath	oath	loathe	the
thy	pith	teeth	Ruth	thong
though	path	tooth	wroth	

(Add other [ð] and [θ] words from ordinary articulation lists, as this is the last glossal compensation.)
Ruth took the oath.
They thought the tooth was loose.
The dentist was loathe to pull my teeth.
Wrath is bad for my health.
That fruit is all pith.

INDEX

163